advent
in natural
childbirth

Janet Schwegel has a master's degree in linguistics, works as an editor, and is the author of *The Baby Name Countdown*. She is a past president of the Association for Safe Alternatives in Childbirth and does the layout of ASAC's *Birth Issues* magazine. When she became pregnant, she and her husband hired a midwife to provide extra support and knowledge. Although they prepared for either a hospital or a home birth, labor went smoothly and their daughter was born at home.

adventures in natural childbirth

TALES FROM WOMEN ON THE JOYS, FEARS, PLEASURES,
AND PAINS OF GIVING BIRTH NATURALLY

Edited and with an introduction by
JANET SCHWEGEL

Foreword by PAM ENGLAND, CNM, MA

Illustrations by CATHY McMILLAN

MARLOWE & COMPANY
New York

Adventures in Natural Childbirth:
*Tales from Women on the Joys, Fears, Pleasures, and Pains
of Giving Birth Naturally*

Copyright © 2005 by Janet Schwegel on behalf of the authors
Foreword copyright by Pam England

Published by
Marlowe and Company
An Imprint of Avalon Publishing Group Inc.
245 West 17th Street • 11th Floor
New York, NY 10011

AVALON
publishing group incorporated

The information in this book is intended to help readers make informed decisions about their
health and the health of their loved ones. It is not intended to be a substitute for treatment by or
the advice and care of a professional health care provider. While the author and publisher have
endeavored to ensure that the information presented is accurate and up to date, they are not
responsible for adverse effects or consequences sustained by any person using this book.

Library of Congress Control Number: 2005921085

ISBN 1-56924-368-9

9 8 7 6 5 4 3 2 1

Book design by India Amos
Printed in the United States of America

Contents

~

Foreword

～

PAM ENGLAND

S TORYTELLING, THE OLDEST form of teaching, is almost a lost art. Only a few generations back, our culture turned a deaf ear to elder story-tellers who once taught and initiated the youth through stories. Still, every-body loves a good story, especially a pregnant woman who yearns for personal guidance from anyone with experience.

The first birth story we hear in our magical childhood years may tune our ears for hearing birth stories later in life, inadvertently creating an invisible fil-ter that allows familiar concepts in and blocks out others. Is it possible to hear a birth story with beginners' mind, to feel it touch us, without measuring it against what we know or believe?

In the film *Big Fish*, Edward Bloom (played by Albert Finney) is a salesman and father who spins lively yarns about his experiences as a young man. His adult son Will (played by Billy Crudup), never knows for sure where truth ends and embellishment begins. Over time he grows frustrated, even embarrassed, by his father's stories. In pursuit of "reality," Will spurns his aging father and discounts his autobiographical anecdotes. At his father's funeral he actually meets the people his father described—and discovers to his surprise that there was a kernel of truth in those stories.

Birth stories are often *Big Fish* stories: they are eternally provocative and rarely objective, and facts are interwoven with sentiment. Who can resist projecting at least a little of their own interpretation or values onto a birth story? It's virtually a sport, and we cheer for, or rail against, the heroes and the villains! It is too easy, even lazy, to get caught up hastily agreeing or disagreeing with a story because it is or isn't in alignment with your values or brings to mind something you are hope to avoid. Instead of responding emotionally to what seems to be the most apparent message, wait!

With deep listening and reflection, many birth stories can have personal meaning for you beyond what may have been presented by the storyteller. Practice listening more deeply. Sit quietly. Be willing to hear a story that may knock an old idea off the shelf. After all, the essence of hearing birth stories is to learn, which means you take in a new idea that at least temporarily rearranges the patterns in your mind. This kind of learning expands and empowers you because it allows you to see, hear, and feel differently.

Reading these birth stories may not only prepare you for your upcoming experience but may also heighten your desire to be conscious of the power of your words when you tell your own story.

Best wishes,
Pam England

PAM ENGLAND, CNM, MA, a registered nurse and certified nurse midwife, developed the "birthing from within" approach in a series of birthing classes designed to help mothers reclaim and celebrate the spiritual, emotional, and psychological aspects of birth as a rite of passage. The coauthor of *Birthing from Within*, England lives in Albuquerque, New Mexico.

Introduction

⌒

JANET SCHWEGEL

W HEN DEE DEE Kopchia was expecting her baby, many times people told her to "just ask for the epidural, morphine, or other forms of pain relief....[W]hy would you go through the pain of natural childbirth?" But Dee Dee said she was "bound and determined that I was not having any drugs whatsoever."

Why not take the drugs and medical treatments that are available to help with labor and delivery? You can even choose to have an elective caesarean section and avoid labor altogether. Why shouldn't you do that? Why strive for a natural childbirth? According to Dr. Jan Christilaw, past president of the Society of Obstetricians and Gynecologists of Canada, the short answer is that "the best birth is an unmedicated vaginal birth."[1]

Most people attempt natural childbirth because they understand that it's better for the mother or for the baby. But natural childbirth is also better for fathers and, it turns out, for society as a whole. *Adventures in Natural Childbirth* is a collection of stories and essays about what can happen when someone sets out to have a natural childbirth. Through the essays and the provocative foreword by midwife Pam England, you'll learn about the the experience and the benefits of natural childbirth through these stories. Even the captions for the illustrations are educational.

Natural childbirth means labor and delivery without pain medication and with as little medical intervention as possible. In her essay introducing the section on birthing naturally with a physician, Dawn Freeman points out that "natural childbirth isn't when you do nothing to prepare for the birth; on the contrary, it happens only when you do many things to prepare." Natural childbirth isn't just an event—it's an attitude. As you read the birth stories in *Adventures in Natural Childbirth*, notice how the mother's confidence level correlates with her achievement of a natural childbirth.

～❧～

Disadvantages of natural childbirth

THERE ARE DISADVANTAGES to natural birth. For one, it can be arduous. After much preparation, planning, and hoping for a natural birth, mothers may feel discouraged when their work results in slow progress in the baby's movement toward the outside world. Birth stories in this book describe some methods of encouraging labor, such as following the advice of a midwife, doula, or nurse to change positions or to vocalize in a different way. Another way to avoid discouragement is to minimize the number of cervical checks. Constant worry about how dilated she is does not help the mother relax and achieve the level of focus that she needs. In fact, cervical checks during labor are not absolutely required. Some caregivers, especially ones who know their clients well, determine progress just by paying attention to the laboring woman and monitoring the baby's heartbeat.

It also helps to know that it's normal and common to feel discouraged during transition, the time when the uterus shifts from pulling to open the cervix to pushing the baby down. In this case, a mother's concerns about her ability to complete the task may be a positive signal of progress. For example, during labor Charlotte Russell, who was training to become a midwife, experienced difficulty and discomfort. When she was ready to push, she didn't want to. Instead, at this point she "contemplated asking the midwives to transport me to the hospital for a C-section." She reports that things were so bad she got nasty with the midwives and yelled at her husband.

Natural childbirth can also be painful. Occasionally women find it excruciating. More often birth stories describe labor as somewhat painful, with feelings of pressure and discomfort. A few women don't feel pain. In particular, watch
for birth stories where the parents train themselves in self-hypnosis, which as
Valerie Larenne states in her birth story "sounds a lot wackier than it is."

Possible complications from vaginal birth include incontinence and bladder prolapse, but surgery is not without complications, either. The risks of C-
sections include infection and hemorrhage in the mother and respiratory
distress syndrome in the baby.[2] Any major surgery requires slow and careful
recovery. As well, women who have had caesareans often regret the fact that they
had difficulty lifting their newborn babies.

A final disadvantage of natural childbirth is its spontaneity. Unlike scheduled Caesarean sections, natural childbirth begins on its own initiative, not necessarily when a mother or a physician finds it convenient. That the timing of
birth may be outside of her control irks some women. But it's the first step in
accepting that when this baby comes, a woman's life is no longer hers alone.

⌒◎⌒

Advantages of natural childbirth

NATURAL CHILDBIRTH EMPOWERS women. It is a life-changing event, and
not just because it produces a baby. It changes a woman's view of her abilities,
reinforcing her belief in her capabilities. After a natural childbirth, many
women feel that they can do anything.

Another bonus of natural childbirth is that the woman's body can bounce
back quickly. The hormones that flow through a woman's body during labor
and delivery help her to recover and bond with her baby. On the other hand,
caesarean sections come with the risks and recovery difficulties of any major
surgery. A big advantage of a natural childbirth over one involving surgical
intervention is that the mother may hold her baby immediately after birth,
sometimes for half an hour or more before any further procedures take place.

Yes, there can be pain involved in labor and delivery, but it's "pain with a purpose." Besides, the human body has an effective way of coping with pain: it
produces endorphins. In their birth stories, a number of mothers note that they
lost track of time or felt sleepy. That might be because they're exhausted from

working hard for a long time, but it's also possible that endorphins were making them sleepy. During my own labor, I felt like I was falling asleep in the pauses between pushes. I wasn't especially tired, and I hadn't missed a night's sleep; it was endorphins taking me to a space between awake and asleep.

Natural childbirth is often more satisfying for partners as well. As Reiko Jodi Halperin notes, "My husband was elated that he was a part of such an awesome experience. He felt like a participant in his daughter's delivery instead of a bystander in the room."

In the essay introducing birthing naturally with a doula, Tracey Stolarchuk states: "Natural childbirth should definitely be more commonplace. The natural process of birth through hormonal changes prepares babies for transition outside the womb, facilitates bonding between mothers and babies, and prepares women for the tasks of motherhood."

Most important, however, natural childbirth allows the hormones that have been working for women for thousands of years to fulfill their functions. This is more important than just helping a woman through labor and delivery. Birth-related hormones also affect well-being much later in life. Dr. Michel Odent's research into primal health, the lifelong effects of how we are born, reveals a correlation between non-normal childbirth and suicide, violence, drug addiction, and autism. Dr. Odent, a renowned obstetrician and author, credited with introducing the concepts of home-like birthing rooms and birthing pools, believes that more childbirth without interference would benefit Western societies.

Birthing naturally with hormones

THE HORMONES OXYTOCIN, endorphins, and adrenaline are produced during natural childbirth. The first two promote labor; the latter inhibits it.

Oxytocin, which helps us feel good and triggers nurturing feelings and behaviors, increases gradually during pregnancy and sharply during labor, stimulating contractions. Low levels of oxytocin cause contractions to stop or slow, contribute to excessive bleeding after birth, and therefore often lead care providers to intervene.

Endorphins are pain-relieving hormones that rise steadily and steeply during natural childbirth. High endorphin levels can produce an altered state of consciousness that helps women flow with the birthing process even when it is long and arduous, leaving them alert, attentive, and even euphoric after birth, thus strengthening the mother-infant relationship. Endorphin levels drop sharply with the use of epidurals and some analgesics such as morphine.

Feeling fearful or threatened during labor may cause the production of adrenaline, the "fight or flight" hormone. Its effect on laboring women is to slow or stop labor as well as to increase the mother's sense of panic and pain.

A woman can promote the production of oxytocin and endorphins and reduce the production of adrenaline by:

- staying calm, comfortable, confident, and relaxed
- avoiding disturbances, such as unwelcome people or noise
- staying upright, because the pressure of the baby against the mother's cervix and pelvic floor stimulates oxytocin
- engaging in nipple stimulation before birth and allowing the baby to suckle immediately afterward, because these actions increase oxytocin
- avoiding an epidural or morphine for pain control
- being informed and prepared
- trusting her body and her capability to birth
- trusting her caregivers
- being in a calm, peaceful, and private environment
- avoiding intrusive, painful, disruptive procedures[3]

~~~

Reality childbirth

IN OUR CULTURE, people who aren't directly involved in birthing care typically don't know much about birth. How many births have you witnessed? Probably none other those of your own children. Compare that to the number of births you know of, the number of friends and family members you know who have had children. Births happen all the time, but we rarely see them firsthand.

Things used to be different. As Claudia Villeneuve points out in her essay introducing the section on birthing naturally with a doula, "When a woman went into labor, it was expected that other women in her community would come to her home and help. This was a typical social expectation that had the added benefit of exposing childless women to the experience of birth."

Many of our notions about birth come from mass media such as television, where birth is often portrayed as a terrifying experience in which women end up with their feet in the air, surrounded by people who are yelling at them to push. In her birth story Angela Miller says, "From the time I found out I was pregnant, I wanted to have a natural birth. I have never been more determined and more scared about anything in my life. Why the fear? Sadly enough, there is so much negativity surrounding birth, especially in the United States. I had bought into those notions my whole life, almost to the point where I didn't know if I wanted to have children. I knew that birth was going to be the hardest thing I would ever do, especially if I was going to do it naturally."

Adventures in Natural Childbirth provides realistic portrayals of births.

❧

The organization of
Adventures in Natural Childbirth

BECAUSE THE SINGLE most important factor in trying to achieve a natural childbirth is choice of caregiver (followed by choice of birth setting), *Adventures in Natural Childbirth* is divided into sections by type of caregiver situation: birth with a midwife, birth with a physician, birth with a doula, and birth without assistance (unassisted birth). (These sections are based on choice of birth care. There's no section on birthing with a nurse because one does not normally have a choice of nurses.) Each section begins with an essay on how different types of caregivers can help a woman achieve her goal of natural childbirth. The introductory essay is followed by birth stories, first-person accounts of pregnancy, labor, and delivery.

Adventures in Natural Childbirth contains a variety of birth stories: some women are calm and relaxed while some women are panicky; some births are exhilarating and painless while some births are excruciating; some births are completely natural, even unattended by medical personnel, while some births end with epidurals and caesarean sections; sometimes waters break early, sometimes waters break late; sometimes labor is short, sometimes it's long; sometimes being in water provides great relief to the mother, sometimes it provides no relief; some babies are born at home, some are born in a birth center or at a hospital—one baby is even born on the way to the hospital; and so on. Some stories are detailed blow-by-blow accounts; others are hazy evocations.

BIRTHING NATURALLY WITH A MIDWIFE

Midwives specialize in natural childbirth. They're trained in the normal processes of birth, in coping methods, and in recognizing trouble signs. Midwives are typically restricted from performing medical procedures to intervene in the course of labor or delivery. The restrictions vary depending on the local regulations. For example, in her birth story Karin Keogh explains that the midwives at the birth center couldn't give Pitocin (oxytocin) during labor because that is an intervention in the course of labor, but they could give it afterward to stop bleeding.

Midwives may not do some of the things that doctors may, but the routine tests that physicians and midwives perform during prenatal visits are the same: proteins and sugar in urine, the size of the fundus, and the baby's heartbeat. The difference is that doctors may check the urine sample without announcing the result, whereas midwives are more likely to explain to the mothers how to read the stick and let the mothers check their urine themselves. Midwives can even order laboratory tests like blood tests and chorionic villae sampling to check for chromosomal abnormalities. Unlike physicians, however, midwives typically spend half an hour to an hour with a client at each prenatal visit.

Studies have repeatedly shown that births attended by midwives are as safe as or safer than those attended by physicians. For an example, see Dr. Marsden Wagner's article titled "Midwifery in the industrialized world," which summarizes numerous studies, concluding: "scientific evidence proves that: midwives are as safe or safer than doctors for primary maternity care; using midwives greatly reduces the rates of unnecessary obstetrical interventions; midwifery services lead to considerable cost savings; midwives have more success in reaching socially disadvantaged groups; women have more satisfaction with midwife-managed care."[4]

Perhaps because midwives typically get to know a woman and her family well, women report high levels of satisfaction with the care they receive from midwives. Midwives aren't saints, though. Sometimes they have disagreements with their clients. For example, Lanna Palsson is pressured by her midwife to agree to a hospital birth, although she avoids the hospital in the end. As midwifery becomes more common in North America, complaints about midwives will surely increase. To avoid finding yourself in that situation, research your midwife well, just as you would any important care provider.

BIRTHING NATURALLY WITH A PHYSICIAN

While it's true that midwives specialize in natural birth and that physicians practice medical births for the most part, it is possible to have a natural childbirth in a hospital with a physician. In her introduction to the section on birthing naturally with a physician, Dawn Freeman points out that the mother has to be informed and determined, and the physician must be enlightened. Dawn encourages women to shop around for such a physician.

Some women, like Angela Miller, feel safer in hospital. It's important that a woman be in a place where she feels safe when she is in labor. If that safe place is a hospital, that's fine.

A number of the stories in the physician and doula sections also show that the mother has to be willing to stand up to the authority of the hospital staff, not an easy thing to do when one is vulnerable or when labor is progressing slowly. A number of the mothers flatly refuse to cooperate with some of the demands of the hospital staff. Dee Dee Kopchia, for example, resists repeated offers of an epidural and pressure to sign an epidural waiver. Mothers need to know that they are in control of their bodies and their births. They have the right to refuse care that isn't required.

Achieving a natural childbirth in a hospital is particularly tricky if the mother's water breaks before contractions begin. To avoid complications, physicians establish a deadline of twenty-four or thirty-six hours from time of water breaking to time of birth. This timeline, and the fact that labor is obviously about to begin, pressures the parents to go to the hospital early. Once at the hospital, the mother will probably have a fetal monitor attached and other interventions may be offered. In general, the more time a mother spends in labor at the hospital, the more likely it is that she won't have a natural childbirth.

It's important that women do have natural childbirths with physicians and nurses in hospitals. When women give birth naturally within the medical system, it improves the system: hospitals develop ways to facilitate natural birth, and staff learn how to make birthing families comfortable and help birthing women achieve their goals.

BIRTHING NATURALLY WITH A DOULA

Birthing assistants, more commonly known as doulas, can aid parents tremendously in following their birth plans. Besides providing emotional support and suggesting ways to cope with contractions, doulas can help mothers deal with hospital procedures. While doulas cannot make decisions about care—the mother or father has to give the approval or refusal for any procedure—their perspective and presence can alleviate some of the pressure that parents may feel.

In the chapter introducing the section on birthing naturally with a doula, Claudia Villeneuve presents scenarios in which nurses and physicians offer interventions to mothers whose birth plans indicate that they want natural births. For example, when offered an epidural for the pain, "the mom says she wants a natural birth. The nurse replies that this is fine but that an epidural will give her a chance to sleep. The mom looks at the doula, and the doula asks if she wants the epidural or if she wants some time to think about it. The mom says she needs time to think about it, and the nurse leaves."

A number of the doula birth stories describe short labors, possibly because the parents hired a doula to help them after having an unsatisfactory birth experience. Since this is not the mother's first experience of labor, with the confidence of the doula, the mother labors quickly. In addition, a number of the birth stories in the doula section involve vaginal birth after caesarean (VBAC), possibly because such births often take place in a hospital but the mother hires a doula to help avoid another caesarean.

BIRTHING NATURALLY UNASSISTED

As Christina Otterstrom-Cedar explains in the introductory chapter to the section on birthing naturally without assistance (unassisted birth), people step further outside the mainstream for a variety of reasons. These people are typically very knowledgeable about and confident in a woman's ability to give birth naturally. You may have a different perspective after reading these stories, most of which describe calm and fulfilling births.

BIRTHING NATURALLY
FOR THE FIRST TIME OR THE NEXT TIME

Finally, Reinekke Lengelle's essay provides insight into dealing with the reality that births don't always go as desired. Reinekke had high expectations for herself before her first birth; she was convinced that nothing other than a natural birth would do. But things turned out otherwise. She has drawn from this experience and from her consulting work to write the final chapter in *Adventures in Natural Childbirth*.

Birthing naturally

EVERY BIRTH IS an adventure. Part of the adventure may be finding out that soaking in a bathtub doesn't alleviate your labor pains. One woman decided that it didn't help much but it was better than being out of the tub.

Many women find going for a walk during labor or walking up and down stairs is effective in positioning their babies, helping them move into the birth canal. Be sure to read Courtney Crow Wyrtzen's description of the walk she took during labor.

Although some women know that they want a natural childbirth long before they are pregnant, sometimes a woman, like Courtney Crow Wyrtzen, experiences a "standard" medical birth and is satisfied with it until she reads a book about birthing in North America. Many women come to natural childbirth after a birth with medical interventions that they later realize may not have been necessary.

Often a book will trigger an epiphany about childbirth. (For further reading, see the list of resources near the end of this book.) There's a lot of growth in these stories, and it doesn't just happen in the mother's belly.

Birthing naturally with a midwife

ANNEMARIE VAN OPLOO

I N ORDER TO birth naturally, a woman has some very basic needs: privacy, security, faith, encouragement, and as little interference as possible, among others. In the philosophy and principles that guide their profession, and in their practice, midwives have always respected these primal needs, thereby facilitating natural birth. In fact, midwives are specialists in normal birth, offering an expertise unlike that of physicians because they view birth holistically.

Choosing a midwife as your primary caregiver and choosing to birth at home in a familiar environment provides you with the best chance for a safe and natural birth—it's a statistical reality! Current research shows that midwives have an excellent record of providing safe and satisfying primary care in homes, hospitals, and birth centers, world wide and locally, with morbidity rates lower than and mortality rates equal to physician care, as well as greatly reduced rates of unnecessary obstetrical interventions.

This chapter defines what a midwife is, the ways in which the midwifery philosophy and the principles of the midwifery model of care help ensure a safe and positive birth experience, and a discussion of the future of midwifery care and natural birth. The way in which we birth affects us all—women, children, families, and communities—at an extremely deep level. The information provided in this chapter and the birth stories that follow reveal the advantages of midwifery care and will, hopefully, inspire you to join in asserting that the care midwives provide should be the standard for child-bearing women everywhere.

◦◦◦

What is a midwife?

THE WORLD HEALTH Organization uses the following definition of a midwife:

> A midwife is a person who ... has acquired the requisite qualifica-tions to ... practise midwifery. She must be able to give the neces-sary supervision, care and advice to women during pregnancy, labor and the postpartum period, to conduct deliveries on her own respon-sibility and to care for the newborn and the infant. This care includes preventative measures, the detection of abnormal condi-tions in mother and child, the procurement of medical assistance and the execution of emergency measures in the absence of medical help. She has an important task in health counseling and educa-tion, not only for the women, but also within the family and the community ... She may practise in hospitals, clinics, health units, domiciliary conditions or in any other service.[1]

Since the beginning of human history and all over the world, women have helped women and their families in the transition to motherhood. There has always been "a tendency to give birth close to their mother, or close to some-body who can play the role of the mother ... This is the root of midwifery. A midwife is originally a mother-figure."[2]

A midwife—the word means "with woman"—was self-sufficient in that she used her eyes, ears, mouth, nose, hands, and heart to assess and assist women and their babies. She carried a wealth of knowledge and experience regarding childbearing and the herbs that could positively influence labor, birthing, postpartum recovery, and breastfeeding. This knowledge was gained from personal experiences; patient, watchful attendance at many births; and the oral teachings of previous generations. Midwives carried few instruments, and those they did carry were mainly tools to help support women during pushing, such as stones, bricks, wooden staffs, and eventually birth stools. They used non-invasive techniques to help nature along only when necessary.

These women were called wise women, earth mothers, and were greatly respected in their communities for their wisdom and expertise. Through their role at births midwives strengthened the connections between generations of women and their families; helping build the foundations of community. This continues today: families who choose midwifery care often establish supportive connections with one another, creating an informal social support network that extends well past the childbearing year.

The midwifery philosophy

SIMPLY PUT, HERE is the philosophy that midwives observe: The practice of midwifery is based on the understanding that pregnancy, labor, and birth are profound experiences that carry significant meaning for a woman, her family, and her community. Midwifery is grounded in the belief that having a baby is a natural life process and an opportunity for considerable growth. The intent of midwifery care is to enhance these life experiences. Midwifery is traditionally holistic, combining an understanding of the social, emotional, cultural, spiritual, psychological, and physical aspects of a woman's reproductive experience. Midwives promote wellness in women, babies, and families both autonomously and in collaboration with other health care professionals.[3]

Childbearing as a normal life process

THE MIDWIFERY PHILOSOPHY regards conception, pregnancy, labor, birth, and breastfeeding as normal, natural processes, not medical events. Beginning in the 1400s, a complex set of historical and social circumstances began the shift in maternity care from midwife to physician, from home to hospital. By the end of the 1800s, the normal processes of childbirth were viewed as a pathology requiring technological intervention in most industrialized countries, and male-dominated physicians and their nursing counterparts controlled the care of childbearing women.

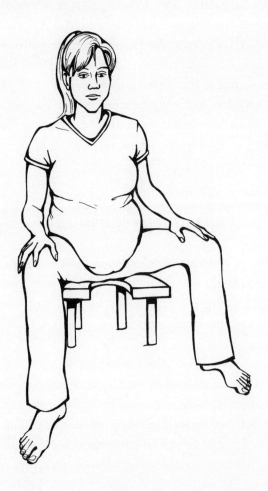

BIRTHING STOOLS OR BIRTHING BENCHES allow a woman to give birth supported in a squat. Birthing stools have been documented in history since the Middle Ages and even became items of interior decoration. They can be fashioned out of small chairs with the seat cut into a U shape or purchased from specialty manufacturers with padding and steel bars. Sitting on a birthing stool allows women to squat for a long time, which is something Western women are not accustomed to because of the common use of tall chairs. Sitting on a birthing stool widens the pelvis and allows more room for the baby's head to pass through. It also relaxes the pelvic floor, which can reduce the chance of perineal tears. Combined with the force of gravity, birthing stools contribute to a gentle vaginal birth without the need for episiotomies, forceps, vacuum, or caesarean sections.

Sarah Day, registered midwife (RM), observes that "women have become dependent on technology and have lost the trust in their own bodies."[4] A midwife today spends time to help a woman reframe her beliefs about birth and her body's abilities so she will regain that trust. Childbirth is a time when a woman's power and strength emerge full force, but it is also a vulnerable time, and a time of many changes presenting opportunities for personal growth. A midwife's trust in these processes helps women merge with their own power in order to realize their potential in childbearing and mothering. They also honor the fear, pain, and work of labor as part of what makes birth a rite of passage. Midwives believe that more than 90 percent of women can and should birth naturally.

As Cathy Harness, RM, simply puts it, "I trust the process God has designed." Women who want a natural birth benefit from having a primary caregiver who truly believes in the process of birth and women's abilities to birth naturally. Pam England, certified nurse midwife (CNM), writes in her bestseller *Birthing from Within* that the ongoing infusion of confidence throughout pregnancy and labor from a midwife is probably the one of the most important ingredients in a natural birth.

✑

Minimal intervention

WE FORGET THAT just a few generations ago the only way to birth a baby was naturally; there were no pharmaceutical, surgical, or technological interventions. There is anthropological and archaeological research that shows that for thousands of years women were trusted to birth without invasive interventions and that the birthing process was women's territory—women were in control of what happened at births. The only thing a woman could do was believe in her ability, trust her body and the process, and birth through the pain and fear she may have felt. No one had told her to doubt; she had seen and heard birth before; she was not ashamed of her body; and she had other women supporting her.

Roxanne Potter, CNM, asserts that "when you create an environment of love, support around you, labor is very cope-able."[5] Midwives take a supportive rather than interventionist role. They see labor through patient eyes and assist in the natural process with a minimal amount of evidence-based intervention only when necessary. Their experience and education have made them specialists in normal childbearing. Midwives are committed to allowing normal physiological processes to unfold without immediately looking for a substitute. The results of an Alberta, Canada, study of comparable low-risk births shows that the rate of caesarean section was two-thirds lower with midwifery care while the rate of other interventions was halved.

~~⌖~~

What sorts of things do midwives use to help ensure a successful natural birth?

FOLLOWING CUES FROM the laboring woman, midwives encourage the use of a variety of techniques that carry no risk and work with a woman's normal physiological processes. Besides creating a feeling of security with their familiar presence, midwives actively support the use of the following techniques to cope with the discomforts of pregnancy, lessen the perception of pain, start labor, make contractions more effective, prevent perineal tears or postpartum hemorrhage, shift or turn a baby, and help women summon the stamina needed during the hard work of labor and birthing.

- quiet/privacy
- low lighting
- patient encouragement
- information
- eating and drinking
- laughter
- heat
- changing positions
- movement (e.g., dancing, walking, lunging)
- music
- massage/massage oils
- visualization
- vocalization (e.g., groaning, moaning, panting)
- sexual play between partners
- nipple stimulation

- masturbation
- warm water (e.g., shower, bath, pool, compresses)
- acupuncture
- herbs
- transcutaneous electronic nerve stimulation (TENS)
- Bach flower essences
- homeopathics
- sterile water injections
- chiropractic care
- no separation of the mother and baby
- attempting breastfeeding as soon after birth as possible
- aromatherapy/essential oils
- incorporation of the woman's spiritual beliefs/practices
- nutritional counseling

Of course, midwives are also trained to use modern equipment, medications, and oxygen to monitor the woman and baby in labor; to do safe and aseptic procedures such as artificial rupture of membranes, cutting the cord, or suturing tears; and to provide resuscitation or administer medications should this be necessary.

Responsibility for health

BIRTH CAN AFFECT us physically, psychologically, emotionally, spiritually, and sexually. With these most intimate parts of ourselves so intricately involved in the maternity cycle, it is important that we maintain as much responsibility and control as possible.[6] Midwives respect an internal locus of control over health rather than an external one, meaning they encourage women themselves to hold the power rather than allowing a health care professional to take control.

The concept of power is key in natural birth. A woman wanting a natural birth needs to take ownership of her body, her baby, and her birth experience. She must adopt the attitude that she is in charge and that what she wants is most important. She has to assert herself and voice her wishes as well as ensure that no one abuses her rights. She has to ask questions and use her critical thinking abilities when assessing the answers she is given. Midwives promote wellness, intrinsic responsibility, and enable "women to develop the understanding, skills, and motivation necessary to take responsibility and control over their own health."[7]

∿

Partners in holistic care

MIDWIFERY CARE IS a partnership based on mutual respect between a midwife and a woman and her family. When midwives approach their clients as equals, the woman's expertise is respected and included in planning her care. Midwifery care is traditionally holistic. This means the social, emotional, cultural, spiritual, psychological, and physical aspects of the childbearing family's experience are all taken into account when the midwife provides care.

Through empathetic woman-to-woman interaction the midwife learns the woman's fears and desires and other aspects beyond the physical, which undoubtedly influence the pregnancy and labor. This holistic understanding of the woman and her environment is extremely valuable as it helps the midwife provide more effective, individualized care, which in turn helps ensure a natural birth. Of course such a partnership and holistic understanding requires time to develop. The average length of a prenatal visit with a midwife is one half to one hour while the average length of a prenatal visit with an obstetrician is six to ten minutes. Since a midwife is fundamentally accountable to her clients, she is highly committed to ensuring their satisfaction.

∿

Principles of the midwifery model of care

THE BELIEF IN childbearing as a normal process, minimal interventions, women's responsibility for their own health, forming a partnership with women, and a holistic approach to care form the philosophy behind the following principles of the midwifery model of care. These principles are about choice and continuity of care. Women want the freedom to choose where they give birth, who is with them, what position they labor and give birth in, and other choices often unavailable under physician care.

The appropriation of birthing by medicine involves a long history of taking control, power, and freedom away from childbearing women. Maintaining a sense of control over their care is an important reason women choose midwives. Without having good information about their choices, women cannot maintain control over their care, take responsibility for making decisions about those choices, or have the freedom and power to ensure that their choices are respected. Essentially, midwives invite women to create their own individual experience. When women seize this opportunity, they usually succeed in having a natural birth.

INFORMED CONSUMER CHOICE

Many believe that the policies, routines, and interventions of physician-managed, hospital-based, and technologically dependent birth are based on scientific evidence. Some of these include not being allowed to eat during labor, limiting who and how many family or support persons can be in the room, having an intravenous needle inserted upon admission, electronic fetal monitoring, induction or augmentation of labor, artificial rupture of membranes, narcotic and epidural use, birthing in the lithotomy position, episiotomy, forceps or vacuum extraction, surgical birth, separation of mother and baby, and/or supplementing baby with formula or glucose water. In reality, research has shown that these measures are far from beneficial, except in rare situations with true complications.

Sometimes it's scary to question the mainstream approach and act on our own instincts and desires, but "if a woman makes the choice to take an active, decision-making role in her care during pregnancy, birth and postpartum, and demands respect for her choices—she has taken the opportunity to create change—both personally and globally."[8] Informed consumer choice is all about women taking responsibility for making knowledgeable decisions about their care. In order to make knowledgeable decisions, women need to know about their full range of choices in care as well as the nature, benefits, and risks of each alternative. They need to know that they can refuse alternatives presented to them and that they can change their minds at any time.

Every health care professional must follow a code of ethics that respects these rights of the health care consumer. Midwives in particular strive to educate and facilitate informed client decision making rather than have clients blindly follow generalized recommendations. Midwives have no standing orders. Without questioning a woman's right or ability, fear mongering, withholding information, providing biased information, or coercing or pressuring, midwives assist their clients in making truly informed decisions about their care and support them in those choices. This is important to women desiring natural birth. The choice of primary caregiver and the choice of birth setting are two of the most fundamental decisions women make that influence the outcomes of their birth experiences.

CHOICE OF PRIMARY CAREGIVER

In North America it took only a few generations for the shift from midwives as primary caregivers to the majority of births occurring in hospitals with physicians providing care to occur. "In the early years of the twentieth century, midwifery in the United States and Canada was eliminated as a legitimate health profession,"[9] driving midwives underground.

Today, increasing numbers of North American women are choosing midwives. The American national average of babies born into the hands of midwives is 7.4 percent, although in some states it is as high as 20 percent. The Canadian Medical Association reports that 20 percent of Canadian women would like to receive care by a midwife, whether at home or in hospital, and that figure may be even larger. In the Canadian provinces where midwifery care is currently publicly funded, Registered Midwives are in high demand. More and more women are beginning to recognize that midwives can best meet their needs for maternity care. The right to choose a midwife as primary caregiver needs to be respected.

Unfortunately, in North America a hospital birth with a physician as primary caregiver is the only option known to many women and in most places in Canada and the United States virtually the only accessible option. This prevents women from choosing midwifery care and having the best chance to birth naturally.

Choice of birth setting

"It's important that families choose their site of birth ... Women need to labor and birth where they feel safest and most comfortable,"[10] says Meryl Moulton, RM. The options include hospital, home, or freestanding birth center. Midwives respect a woman's right to make an informed choice about the setting for her baby's birth.

Historically, most children were born at home, allowing women to witness birth before having their own children. With this experience no longer available to women, most have little knowledge about birth and harbor all sorts of fears and misconceptions. Therefore, they often make the mistaken assumption that a hospital is safest place to birth and make an uninformed choice. "Women who go to the hospital for safety don't realize that they're giving up a great deal of safety for themselves and their babies ... The percentage of women who actually need to be in a hospital ... is very small."[11] Hospitals are designed to care for acutely ill people; being pregnant, being in labor, and birthing are not illnesses. Even if you enter a hospital under the care of a midwife or an enlightened physician, the institution still reflects many of our cultural values: hierarchical relationships, cleanliness, time, dependence on technology, control over nature, and dissociation from the body. No matter how well-informed and well-intentioned she may be, these often undermine the birthing woman's focus, power, confidence, sense of self, and determination to have a natural birth.

Women often find more satisfaction in a freestanding birth center offering care based on the midwifery model. Births centers don't just strive to provide a home-like atmosphere; the midwifery model of care is reflected in the centers attitudes and policies. There are very few birth centers in Canada, but they are more common in the United States, where almost 100 freestanding birth centers are spread across 32 states.

At home women don't have to worry about unnecessary interventions or exposure to foreign pathogens and are able to remain focused on labor. Having to leave the familiarity of home during labor to go to another birth facility is often the beginning of hindering the normal progress of labor. "Women ... have chosen to give birth at home for many generations. Available scientific evidence demonstrates that planned home birth with midwives is a safe and viable option for healthy low-risk women ... Home birth should be an available option for all childbearing women."[12] Home is the best place to ensure a natural birth.

CONTINUITY OF CARE

According to Sharyne Fraser, RM, continuity of care—having one caregiver throughout the process—is the most critical aspect of midwifery. Midwives offer comprehensive continuity of care throughout the childbearing cycle. This means a woman receiving midwifery care can receive preconception counseling; prenatal care including testing, ultrasound, and lab work; prenatal preparation; labor support; care during and after the birth; breastfeeding support and postpartum follow-up all through the same caregiver. In addition, the midwife is on call twenty-four hours a day.

Continuity allows the midwife and the woman to get to know each other and establish a friendship that often lasts beyond the childbearing year. Midwives get to know their clients quite well, which improves their ability to assess their clients' well-being and helps them detect concerns, potential risks, and problems more quickly than fragmented mainstream medical care could. "Although continuity of care is facilitated through a one to one relationship between a midwife and her client, midwifery care can be provide by a small group of midwives if the client has the opportunity to establish relationships with all the members of the group."[13] Continuity ensures that only familiar faces will be present at the birth, so women feel more secure.

Outside of the midwifery model of care a woman may receive care from many different people and institutions. An obstetrician chosen as primary caregiver usually has only brief contact with a woman during her labor and is often not the one actually there for the birth. A lack of continuity in caregivers sharing this significant time in a woman's life can result in a feeling of confusion and isolation.

"Research supports the importance of keeping the same caregiver(s) for pregnancy, labor, and birth. Continuity of care leads to less drug use in labor, shorter labors, and babies less likely to need resuscitation at birth. Parents also feel more satisfied."[14]

~∽∾⌢

The future: midwifery care and natural birth

BIRTH IS THE sacred beginning, the root of everything. By putting birthing women and babies in the center of care, by respecting their wisdom, and by honoring and trusting the normal physiological, psychological, emotional, social, and spiritual process of birth, midwives ensure that women have the best chance at a natural birth without unnecessary interventions. In natural birth women can create a sacred, calm, loving, trusting environment around themselves and their babies. They may come out of the experience having regained a sense of trust in their instinctual wisdom and with a confidence that strengthens them as mothers.

"Midwifery is an essential profession," Ina May Gaskin, certified professional midwife (CPM), says. "A midwife's work means something: it prepares the woman to go through childbirth in a way that's transformative and empowering. The empowerment and self respect she learns in labor is passed on to the child in a loving relationship."[15] Childbearing, childrearing, and being born into the world surrounded by these positive qualities helps prevent feelings of fear, mistrust, shame, and alienation. Midwifery care that facilitates natural birth is the path toward a kinder, gentler, nonviolent world. Midwives give us hope for the future, help us fulfill our vision of natural birth as the norm, validate the home environment as a vital force in our lives, and the special nature of their care of birthing women and babies influences the fabric that binds us together as human beings.

~∽∾⌢

What vision do we hold for the future of midwifery?

TODAY IN NORTH AMERICA we have two diametrically opposed models for maternity care: the medical model and the midwifery model. In order to ensure a better future for natural birth and midwifery, the principles of mid-wifery care/midwifery model should be respected in the broader maternity services context. If they are not, it means childbearing women will continue to have their choices restricted and care dictated to them.

The midwifery model is also cost-effective in the long and short term, but as Dr. Marsden Wagner, former World Health Organization regional officer for women's and children's health, warns, "Change won't come easy. It's all about territory. It's about power. It's about control. And at the end of the day, it's about money."[16]

In the Dutch model of childbirth, midwives are the gatekeepers of maternity care. Care is publicly funded and midwives and physicians work together in a way that provides the most effective care. In fact, only midwifery care is reimbursed by Dutch insurance, unless a woman is referred to an obstetrician for a medical condition. A woman choosing obstetrician care without a med-ical reason must pay out of pocket.

In the Dutch model natural birth and home birth are actively supported. Physicians receive training from midwives in normal birth, and physicians do not receive extra payment for specific obstetrical interventions or for per-forming surgical births, which may explain their low intervention and cae-sarean rates.

> In the Netherlands, over a third of all births are planned home births with a midwife in attendance, and the number of planned home births is slowly rising. Another third of births are midwife-attended hospital births. Maternal and perinatal mortality rates are equal to or better than rates in other industrialized countries. The national Caesarean section rate is nine percent. Nearly every Dutch obstetrician supports the present system, and in 1997, the National Government gave the Dutch Midwifery Association 10 million guilders [5.6 million U.S. dollars] for the further promo-tion of midwifery and planned home birth.[17]

An optimum maternity care system in North America will require midwives and the midwifery profession to have equal standing with physicians and the medical profession. A challenge will be to maintain the qualities of authentic midwifery care within such a system. In a conversation with Cathy Harness, RM, she emphasized that "the simple, sweet, woman-to-woman aspects of traditional midwifery must not be lost" in the evolution of the midwifery profession. In schools of midwifery, and under regulation, midwives are being trained to follow policies and protocols established by or to appease the medical establishment. "They feel they are prisoners of a system and that the system is destroying the art of midwifery. Some of them just stop working, others try to fight the system from the inside to no avail ... A midwife is supposed to be a wise woman. Being a wise woman is the opposite of being a narrow technician."[18] Maybe we can find a vision for the future of midwifery world wide in the Dutch model for natural birth.

Perhaps an over-eagerness to attain legitimacy within the established health care system has led to the unfortunate. "What is happening is that my model of care doesn't fit easily with regulated midwifery," lamented Barbara Scriver, RM, in conversation recently. Midwifery care in some industrialized nations has already been usurped by the medical model and no longer reflects the authentic roots of the midwifery model. Only if we demand natural birth within an authentic midwifery model of care can we reverse this trend, for the future of natural birth and true midwifery care are intertwined. Pam England, CNM, in her lecture *The Truth About Childbirth*, declares that we are all grieving birth in this culture. We need to explore the issues surrounding birth and the treatment of women and babies at the beginning of life. Whether we like it or not these are political issues, not just personal ones. "If, through fear or ignorance, we ... allow technocracy to take over, woman-centered childbirth may be lost forever."[19]

ANNEMARIE VAN OPLOO holds a Bachelor of Science degree in nursing from the University of Alberta, a certificate in human resources and labor relations from Athabasca University, and is a certified doula with DONA International. She is the mother of two children, both born at home with midwives attending. For her birth stories visit www.birthissues.org. A passionate advocate for midwifery care and de-institutionalizing birth, Annemarie provides doula care specifically for midwifery clients and lively educational sessions on a variety of topics related to birthing. She has sat as the consumer representative on the Alberta Midwifery Health Disciplines Committee and is a long time member of the Alberta Association for Safe Alternatives in Childbirth (ASAC), contributing regularly to their publication *Birth Issues* since 1995. She is also a member of the Writers' Guild of Alberta.

Kari Jones's birth story

It is almost birth time.

I know because I dream about it every night. In sweaty dreams, candles flicker, water boils, and I groan as wind blows through the cracks in our creaky house. I always wake, panting, before the dream baby is born.

"I can do it," I think as I lie cooling off, my duvet thrown down to the foot of the bed. I turn to look at Michael, tucked under his covers, and when he responds to my motion by rolling over to cuddle me, I push him away. I can feel every hair on his body, his own heat against mine. I stand, take a trip to the bathroom, pour cool water over my face.

During the day at work, in the middle of a conversation about the rainforest, my tummy ripples. Hands stretch out to touch. We laugh. But then those muscles contract, and I find it hard to move, to reach over to look at another book to see what they have said about the rainforest.

It is almost birth time. I know because every time I move, my muscles contract and my stomach hardens like rock. I walk slowly. I think slowly. Time slows.

I dream again. Steaming candles, groaning wind. In the middle of this night, an ocean opens and water fills my bed.

"It has started," I tell Michael. His sleep-fuzzied mind doesn't believe me until he reaches over to my side of the bed and feels the water. As in a dream, we stumble out of bed and put down the plastic sheet we bought on our midwife's advice to protect the bed. Not quite believing, we fall back into bed and sleep in fitful dreams. Through the night my body hardens and groans and my mind wonders one last time what it will be like.

It is morning and someone has called the midwife and our friend Laurie, who will come. It must have been Michael who called; it wasn't me. I was groaning in silence on the bed, then in the bathroom, covered by a blanket since clothes were too uncomfortable. I pace around the apartment, stop while contractions take hold of my mind and grip it with a fierceness I have never encountered.

"Hold a vision of a challenge you overcame," the midwives told me long before I was in labor. I picture myself at the top of a rapid, my kayak bouncing underneath me, my mouth wide open as I yell in terror and exhilaration. I envision navigating the waves until I am out the other side, shouting still, this time in joy. The contraction lets me go. I breathe and wait for the next one.

Michael is behind me, pushing his own body weight into my back. It is never enough, never quite stops the incessant crushing of muscle in my back. Someone else tries but I say, "No, it must be Michael"; he is the only one strong enough. Though it is not enough, it is better. Bearable.

We pace around and around. Someone offers me orange juice, which I drink greedily, then throw up quickly. My body contracts; I stop moving again. They are faster now, or harder, or both. I can't tell the time between them anymore. It seems like a constant stream. Just as I have brought my mind back from one contraction, the other starts. I can feel my body open, centimeter by centimeter, as the baby moves at its glacial pace.

Time passes. My mind has gone elsewhere to a place where the only passing is of contractions. I ask and am surprised to hear that it is noon. Weren't we greeted by the dawn a few minutes ago?

I am growing tired. I am not sure I can endure this back labor any longer. Michael leans all his weight and strength into every contraction, but it is not enough. The midwife suggests walking down the stairs to turn the baby around, but I can't. I can't. But I do. I cling to Michael and step down, down, down the long flight, then turn around and walk up, up, up until, at the top, the contractions change and my back begins to rest. Later they tell me that walk down and up the stairs took me an hour.

I have had enough now and want to stop for a while, but my body is determined.

"You can endure anything for these hours," I tell myself. I tell myself I am strong. Somewhere outside me I hear voices saying the same thing.

At some point the laboring is over and the pushing begins. I have no control over this. My body happens. My mind goes along. I am relieved at first, then discover that the pushing is harder than the laboring. I lean into it, groan with a noise from deep inside my chest, grip Michael with a strength that takes him by surprise. Later he jokes he must have endured as much pain as I did, and I can't quite say no when I see the deep bruises along his side from my inhuman grip.

I push and groan, push and groan. I walk slowly toward the bed. On the way, I almost give up until the midwife's voice penetrates my mind. "I am not going to let you have this baby in the middle of the hallway. Get up and walk to the bed. You can do it."

I walk more. I push and push and groan a deep down sound until my body bursts and time stands still. The baby has crowned, and the moment has come.

That brief moment becomes the most fear filled in my life as I realize that there is no turning back. I notice the orange daisies, placed so carefully in a blue glass next to the bed. The orange is strong. It swallows the fear and I decide the time has come. I take a deep breath, look up at Michael, and push.

The baby is born.

"It is over," I think. The long months of pregnancy are gone. I laugh, feeling light, then turn my still lumbering body over to look at my baby in the bed. It is a boy. How strange. We thought he was a girl.

He bawls and bawls. We laugh. "He is excited to see us," we say. He cries and cries, his purple body sprawled on the bed as hands caress and hold him. The midwife uses a small syringe to pull muck out of his mouth, wipes his eyes and ears, takes a quick look to see if all is there, as it should be.

Michael picks him up carefully, this wobbly bundle, and places him on my lap under my overlarge breasts. I breathe deeply and realize that I am hungry, having missed breakfast and lunch. The baby is hungry, too, and mouths for my breast. I try to hold him to me, to let him place his mouth on my nipple but cannot. His body turns one way and his head another. His arms flail. I laugh, still stunned by the labor, still attached to this baby by the umbilical cord.

The midwife lets us lie for a few minutes then asks Michael to cut the cord. She hands him a pair of scissors and he snips a few inches away from the baby. Then my body contracts again and the placenta comes out in a gush of blood. The midwife holds it up for us to see. "That is where he lived all this time." We laugh. Laurie leans in and strokes the baby's face.

The midwife shows Michael and Laurie how to swaddle the baby. I am too tired, too sore to watch. I lie for a moment, then hold the baby and try to feed him again.

This time it works. His lips open wide, and he sucks with a pull I never expected until the colostrum rushes through my breast to his mouth. How does this baby have so much power in his tiny mouth?

Someone brings me a banana. I eat. I hold the baby in his swaddling clothes, resting while others talk. "It was so amazing when we could see the baby's head." "I am so glad Kim suggested walking down the stairs." "Wow, you almost had that baby in the hallway." "You were so brave, so strong." I don't remember the moments they speak of. It is already a dream.

A few minutes later in the bath, I forget that there is a baby, remember just that I am not pregnant any more. Someone else is holding him, laughing in excitement. I only know that my body isn't heavy any more, that I am thirsty, hungry, tired, sore.

Later, in the night, when Michael and I are taking turns sleeping, the baby's eyes look up at me. The orange daisies are no longer needed.

His fingers caress me with their whisper touch. My body cries through blood, milk, and tears.

He is mine. And I am his forever more.

≪᠗≫

ROBIN JOHNSON'S BIRTH STORY

I CAN HEAR my midwife, Joanna, repeat it over and over again in slow, soothing tones: "Strong and powerful woman. Strong and powerful woman." It's an odd thing for someone to be saying to me, I think. Yet her words are like the warmth of the water I am squatting in, and they soak in.

I am surrounded by love: by my mom, Lorraine, one of the strongest women I know; and by Kaare, my husband, best friend, and greatest love.

I never thought I'd be in this place, at least not in this state. I had always imagined myself writhing in pain on a hard hospital bed in starched sheets stamped "Property of the Health Department," under humming fluorescent lights. "The professionals" would be scurrying about, tethering me to machines and talking in foreign medical tongues. I had to find another way.

After coming across a copy of *Birth Issues* magazine and reading it cover to cover, I started calling the midwives listed in the directory. They were wonderful to talk to, and I set up appointments to meet a couple of them. It didn't take long for me to recognize a difference in this kind of care and set my heart on it.

I decided upon a new program called shared care maternity, where the midwifery care is shared with a physician and paid for by health care insurance. This program advocates natural birth, a process that does not include the use of drugs or interventions and that presents the option of a water birth. To me, it seemed like the perfect choice. I looked forward to the exceptional care and personal attention the midwives would provide and started to prepare myself for the natural birth I desired.

Every appointment with the two midwives, Joanna and Noreen, confirmed in my mind that this was the best choice I could have made. I was always treated as an active participant, not just a client. I was involved in testing my own glucose and protein levels, monitoring my baby's heart rate, and discussing the progress of my pregnancy. It was wonderful to have a full half hour each appointment to ask all my questions and to talk about my feelings and concerns. I was never made to feel insignificant or silly, could share a tear or laugh, and never left without a warm hug.

Toward the end of my pregnancy, I asked Noreen whether she or Joanna would deliver my baby. She told me that neither of them would. When she saw that I was confused, she clarified by saying that although one of them would be in attendance at the birth, I would be the one doing the delivering. Case in point: Noreen was establishing me as the expert when it came to my own body and birth. It was very strengthening and liberating.

With the birth location and birth attendant chosen, I only had my fears left to face. I think I began to fear childbirth almost as soon as I could understand what it was. I would hear women's horror stories that always seemed to have a fish tale quality to them, and I would question whether or not this was a club I wanted to join one day. There was never any doubt that the actual birth was wonderful and blessed, but the journey to get there always seemed to be portrayed as horrible, so horrible, in fact, that it was best to avoid it, with drugs, induction, caesarean section, whatever, just to get that baby out quickly and with as little pain as possible.

With labor and delivery being treated as an emergency, as a dangerous and fragile situation, it's no wonder that it's hard to face it with anything but fear. Yet a little investigation into natural birth painted a much different picture. What a revolutionary idea: my body was made for this purpose and could be trusted; I could handle childbirth and did not need to have drugs! Was it possible that I could do this? Women who had walked this road were telling me I could, and I was eager to join them.

On Sunday night I started having regular contractions, but after a few hours they subsided. I had an appointment with Joanna on Monday morning, and Kaare took time off from work to accompany me. Joanna checked me and confirmed that, already at three centimeters and easily stretching to five, I was indeed well on my way. She told us to go home and get some rest since we would probably be back later in the day.

I did manage to rest a little, in between my spurts of mad nesting! The contractions started picking up again around noon and I cleaned through them until it became too uncomfortable, at which point my husband was able to convince me to lie down. We called Joanna to let her know how things were progressing and that we'd be seeing her soon.

My mom and sister arrived at my house around suppertime, and shortly after we decided it was time to head to the hospital since the contractions were now about three to four minutes apart.

As soon as I was admitted, the staff wanted me up on the bed, strapped to a monitor, but I had already discovered that lying on my back was not a position that was going to work for me. The nurses were very accommodating and allowed me to labor however I felt I needed to, which was generally kneeling on a cushion against the couch. Kaare rubbed my back and applied counterpressure while my mom reminded me to focus and breathe. They also made sure to refuel me with snacks and drinks between contractions. The nurse came in every half hour to measure the baby's heart rate and got right down on the floor with me to do so. Joanna came in from time to time to check on me and to reassure me, then slipped out to catch a nap since she had already been at work all day and obviously wouldn't be leaving any time soon. (No such thing as shift change on her watch!)

By midnight I was six centimeters dilated and the pain had reached a new level. It was time for the pool. The birthing pool looked basically like a large kiddie pool with high, firm sides and a well-inflated bottom, cheerfully covered with colorful tropical fish in masks and snorkels, smiling and blowing bubbles. I waited in anticipation as my labor nurse, Jacquie, filled up the pool with warm water.

As I immersed myself in the water, my whole body sighed with indescribable relief. The warm water and weightlessness soothed and relaxed my fatigued, tense muscles, so much, in fact, that the next several contractions slipped by unnoticed. It felt absolutely wonderful, and I understood why they call it the midwife's epidural.

The bottom was inflated enough for me to kneel on without hurting my knees, and the sides were firm enough for me to lean against and dangle my arms over the sides or grip tightly. I spent the next several hours in this position, rocking back and forth while Kaare poured cup after cup of warm water down my back. Magnolia candles flickered on the windowsill as the moonlight peeked in.

Together the soft music and slowly lapping water contrasted the storm coursing through my body. I was awash in the rhythm of the moment. I was high on endorphins and the tropical fish seemed to be swimming around me, laughing and urging me onward. The intensity was overwhelming. It was more than pain; it was pure energy.

When I complained to Joanna that this third stage was taking too long, she reminded me that my timing was impeccable. I just had to trust my body and let it happen the way it needed to happen. This allowed me to let go of my fear that things had to follow a preconceived pattern and just let my body do what it needed to do. I pushed and pushed from deep inside and with all that was within me.

Before I knew it, the climax was approaching. As I crested the mountain with one stinging push, a beautiful sphere emerged from my body, and I could see its perfection beneath the surface of the water. For one last split second I second-guessed myself and looked up at Joanna as if to say, "Don't you see? That is the head. Aren't you going to do something?" "Just wait for the next contraction and push," she said. I waited what seemed like an eternity, just watching that beautiful head floating between my legs.

I couldn't wait any longer. Every bone, muscle, nerve, and vein sang together in harmony; moaning and groaning in praise to their Creator. It was not the chorus of chaos that I had feared but a song of strength and of surrender. With one last powerful push out came one shoulder, then the other, and before I knew it, there was another person in the pool with me. Elijah Leif entered the world amidst a sea of calm—warm water, candlelight, soft music—peace.

Time seemed to stop as I stared in wonder at this new being. I was frozen. "Was I dreaming?" "Reach down and pick up your baby," came Joanna's reassuring response. I reached down into the water, scooped up his smooth, slippery body, and held him close. I could feel Kaare's strong arms around me as he looked over my shoulder at his new son and reached out gently to touch his miraculous flesh. Elijah opened up his lungs and sang his announcement to the world, a cry so strong and hearty.

We basked in the warmth of the moment for quite a few minutes, just the three of us, gazing into each other's eyes. We had journeyed to the most majestic place on earth and humbly enjoyed the breathtaking view together. I am grateful that Joanna respected this precious time and let us be.

The miracle of Elijah's birth remains just as beautiful in my memory as it was that day and is confirmed each day with growth and giggles, smiles and squirms. My portrayal of labor and birth as beautiful and miraculous is not meant to discount the pain and work involved; it is, after all, called "labor." It was hard and difficult and insanely painful and there were many times when I wanted to give up, give in, if there had been such a choice. It was, however, a labor of love.

There was also a sense of freedom, freedom from fear. Looking back, I have an odd sort of respect for every piercing contraction that was so purposeful in bringing forth my precious baby boy. The experience I had feared had become a blessing, the journey, as well as the destination a thing of beauty. Who would have ever thought it to be so? Certainly not me, little old me: a strong and powerful woman.

JENNIFER CHIPMAN'S BIRTH STORY

SINCE BEFORE I got married, since before I reached my estimated timeline for children, and since before the beginning of my pregnancy, I wanted to give birth naturally. In almost all things, I strive to live in line with nature: organic food, alternative health care, natural fiber clothing, low consumption of material goods—the list goes on and on. For my yet to be conceived children I cast my imagination out along the same lines: cloth diapers, extended breastfeeding, attachment parenting, natural toys, and natural home birth with a midwife. For our family, choosing a natural birth scenario was a given.

I originally met Barbara when I was serving as a volunteer secretary for a local association that advocated alternatives in childbirth. At that time I was childless, mateless, and without a clear idea of when I would have children, but I knew that I wanted to have a midwife-attended birth, and I wanted to start working to promote midwifery funding in our area. I resigned as secretary when I met my husband, married, and moved away. I left the city to live on an organic farm an hour and a half away.

When Larry and I were courting, I made it quite clear that I intended to give birth naturally and at home. This plan made perfect sense to him as he is very much oriented toward nature himself. The summer after we were married, I started to have maternal urges. I was definitely feeling that I wanted to be pregnant. Then one day in June as I was leaning over in the garden weeding carrots, I heard a name whispered in my ear: Kaelynn.

After this, I starting seriously discussing pregnancy with Larry because I felt strongly that our daughter was ready to be born. We discussed it for a time, saying that if we became pregnant in July we would deliver our baby in April, which is a wonderful time to be pregnant and have a baby. Eventually we decided that our financial circumstances weren't what they should be and that it would probably be best to wait another year or two.

July came, and at the end of the month I didn't menstruate. We were pregnant. I took a stick test, told Larry, called my mother, cried, told Larry's parents, and called Barb.

Our baby was due to be born on April sixth, but I started anxiously antici-pating six weeks before the due date. April sixth came and went, and I started wondering if our wee one would arrive on my birthday, April ninth.

On April eighth, we had our last prenatal visit. I asked our midwife, Barb, to check my cervix for progress. She noted that the baby was posterior and I was not dilated at all. She gave me some homeopathic pulsatilla and advised me to crawl around on my hands and knees and to lie in an exaggerated sideways pose if I wanted to try to move baby into a favorable position.

April ninth dawned. I spent parts of the day reading while on my hands and knees on our exercise mat and taking the homeopathic remedy as suggested. That night our family gathered to celebrate my twenty-fourth birthday. We ate cake with fresh strawberries and whipped cream. I commented on the increas-ing number of Braxton Hicks contractions, and we all wondered when the baby would arrive.

That night after I crawled into bed, a contraction took me. I count this one as my first real contraction. The pain crawled around my lower back and felt a bit sharp compared to the Braxton Hicks contractions. I stayed awake, feeling the contractions, timing them, counting the minutes between. I tried sleeping, but the contractions were just strong enough to keep me from dropping into a sound sleep.

As the night progressed, I started tossing and turning in the bed to try to ease the pain in my lower back with each tightening. On several trips to the bath-room, I noticed bloody mucus. Eventually I gave up on sleep and lay in bed, watching the clock radio.

As the contractions moved closer to each other, I woke Larry. At around six AM, the contractions were only six minutes apart, then spread out again to fifteen to twenty minutes apart. They were definitely irregular and not progressive.

We called Barb at around eight AM and let her know what was happening. She suggested a bath.

I ate breakfast with a hot water bottle against my lower back. This eliminated almost all of the pain of the contractions, which were getting strong enough that I had to ask Larry to rub my lower back through them. I then took a bath, which made the contractions stop, and went to sleep until eleven AM when they started again.

Contractions continued throughout the day, and I diligently kept a record of when they would arrive, sometimes six minutes apart for thirty minutes, then nine minutes apart, then fifteen minutes apart, a gap of twenty minutes and back to six minutes apart—very irregular.

Barb called us at around five PM to check in on us, and I read her our extensive contraction time chart. She said that we could stop keeping track and that we would know when labor was upon us. She suggested another bath as a way to either get some rest or speed things up. At this point I was hoping for some sleep.

After our bath and approximately twenty-two hours into our labor, things started speeding up. While I experienced no real feelings of contractions in the bathtub, I was pretty surprised by their intensity when we got out. Suddenly they were two minutes long and coming one after the other in rapid procession.

As I sat on the bed with Larry, moving through the contractions, I started to cry, not due to pain, although it was painful, but because things were moving: we were approaching the birth of our baby, and the physical changes in my body were causing some release to occur. I called my mom and told her to come as soon as she could; Larry called Barb.

Larry rubbed my back through contractions as I worked my way through them on our bed. After a while, I decided that I would try going to the bathroom since I couldn't remember the last time I went. I labored there for a short while, moaning and toughing it out without back rubbing. I also vomited a couple of times, which was unpleasant. I cried again, afraid that the whole labor would be like this, but luckily it only happened twice.

Once I was able to get up, I moved to a chair and leaned against its back, allowing Larry easy access for rubbing. All of the pain of the contractions remained focused in my lower back throughout the entire labor.

Barb arrived a bit after nine PM and checked me for dilation. I was so relieved to learn I was seven centimeters dilated. My only real worry during the prenatal period was that I wouldn't progress quickly during hard labor. I was elated that my work so far had gotten me to this stage.

My mother and one of my sisters arrived soon after Barb. It seemed to take forever for Barb and my mother-in-law to set up the birth tub and fill it. Finally it was ready to go, and I got in. I had originally wanted Larry in the tub with me as well, but I needed his hands for back rubbing.

The contractions continued to become progressively more intense, and I used moaning as my main method of pain control. It was almost as though I assigned each individual pain sensation a noise and followed it through, following the noise with my mind instead of focusing on the pain, starting new noises as my breath ran out or a new sensation arose. There were a couple of contractions that were particularly hard, so hard that I almost "lost it," but Barb helped me stay on top of those. Between contractions I was able to chat normally and comment on the intensity of the labor. I'll always remember saying, "This really isn't so bad!"

Barb asked me to try to urinate again. I couldn't remember when I had last tried as my concept of time was very fluid and loose. I totally relaxed my urinary sphincter, but it took some time for it to release in the pool. As soon as it did, I felt my water break. "My water broke. The baby's coming!" were my exact words. I was so excited!

In that same contraction, I felt an unbearable urge to push and make low grunting noises. I was relieved to make it to the pushing stage and felt like I could relax at this point, no longer having as much pain between contractions as had been the case earlier.

With each contraction, I pushed only as much as my body demanded of me. I felt very relaxed and in no rush to deliver the baby now that I was at this point. Barb monitored the baby's heartbeat and checked internally for progress. I remember her saying that the baby was only a knuckle deep in my vagina. I felt for her, and the first thing I said was, "It feels like she has a lot of hair!" The baby's wrinkly little scalp felt covered with fur.

Soon we started seeing glimpses of black hair peeking through, and slowly, bit by bit, more of our child's hair was revealed. My mother says that she will always remember our baby's hair waving in the water as it emerged from inside of me.

The baby advanced toward the outside world and retreated, advanced and retreated, until finally the crowning occurred. Wow! That was intense! She stayed in that position for two contractions, not going anywhere, and I stretched and stretched. I put my hand on her head to verify that she was down there but needed to remain focused within myself, so I withdrew my hand after only a brief moment of contact.

I pushed and felt relief. I was so internally focused that I didn't even see her emerge in the mirror! Suddenly I was grabbing her and she was on my chest. A girl! "She's so beautiful and perfect and pink!" Looking back at the birth photographs, I see that she was a bit purpled-bluish, but she looked perfectly pink to me at the time.

Still in the water, we held our new baby girl while she cried, cradling her in our arms. I tried to nurse her, but she wasn't interested, not even that night. We tried to get her to "latch on," but she wanted the instant gratification of sucking on her daddy's finger instead. Fortunately, when she was ready to nurse, she had a strong suck, although my nipples experienced a breaking-in period, with soreness and scabs.

After a while Larry cut the cord, and Barb told me that it was time to pass the placenta. At this point I was very reluctant because I didn't want to push any more, but between the two of us we managed to get it out.

I felt weak after the delivery and getting to the bed was difficult; I felt like my insides were falling out. Suddenly, my big belly was floppy and soft, and walking without that huge weight in front was like learning to walk all over again.

Barb examined me and there was no tearing, only a tiny skid mark. Still, the first time I urinated, it burned. Barb put some mint oil in the toilet to help me that first time.

We chose not to have any eye drops or any vitamin K administered. (The birth had been monitored from time to time with a Doppler, but during the pregnancy Barb had used a wooden horn to monitor the baby's heartbeat. We did not pursue ultrasound or group B strep testing.) Our baby weighed eight pounds six ounces at birth and was twenty-one and a quarter inches long. In total we experienced twenty-two hours of latent labor and four hours of active labor, forty minutes of which consisted of pushing.

I was euphoric after the delivery. The world shrank down to a very small speck of holding the baby and watching her, stroking her little limbs and body. I wasn't very aware of what Barb or the rest of the family were doing, but it was around three AM before Barb headed back to the city. Despite being awake on and off for approximately thirty hours, I was flying high. Larry and I both had a hard time getting to sleep due to the excitement of having a new loved one in our bed, but we eventually drifted off.

We did name her Kaelynn, the name I heard whispered in my ear in the carrot patch. I feel very blessed by our successful birthing experience. I reminisced about it for weeks, relived it every day, in awe of the wonder of the birthing process.

KATHERINE DOMSKY'S BIRTH STORY

IT WAS JUST before six o'clock in the morning when I awoke; a Friday morning, the day that was to be my last day of work before maternity leave. My alarm wasn't due to go off for another half hour, but as I lay, alert and still, I became aware of a funny, achy feeling that was radiating out of my pelvis and lower back, almost like menstrual cramps but a bit different somehow. That this would be my baby's birthday did not occur to me. We still had sixteen days to go before our due date. Didn't everyone say that first babies are always late? Of course, I've never been one to believe what everyone else says.

As I lay there in the quiet light of dawn, I began to consider the possibility that these were actual contractions that I was feeling! They didn't hurt, but they were quite a bit stronger than the Braxton Hicks contractions that I'd felt in recent weeks, and they seemed to be coming every five minutes or so. Beside me my husband slept. I'd been awake now for twenty minutes; long enough to see four or five of these crampings come and go. I had ten more minutes before my alarm went off, before I would get in the shower and begin to get ready to leave for work. I decided to wake him and tell him what was happening.

My news jolted him wide awake, but we were both very relaxed, far more relaxed than I'd ever have imagined we'd be in this situation. In part I think we weren't quite able to digest what was going on. Also we were so at ease with how we'd planned to welcome this baby into our lives that it all felt utterly normal. We lay back together in bed, counting what by now we were calling contractions, listening to the radio.

It's funny how everyday things like morning radio can be surreal when you are possibly awaiting the birth of your first child. Everyone else is proceeding with their day-to-day routine, traffic is picking up, construction is getting in people's way, papers are being bought and read on subway cars ... and you are having a baby.

It seems completely crazy now, but I was still planning to go to work, at least for part of the day. "Early labor can go on for days and days," I explained to Darren, who stared at me in disbelief. "You can't go in to work!" He shook his head in wonder. "You're having a baby!"

I still wasn't convinced that this was the case. Besides, what would it hurt to go to work for the morning to say good-bye and tie up those last loose ends? They'd planned a little party, and wouldn't it be lacking in manners to stay home for a few contractions that would probably start to dwindle down in a few hours? We both agreed that, at the very least, we would call our midwife and let her know what was happening.

Fariba, the most gentle spirit of any I've ever met, was quick to side with Darren and insisted that going to work was out of the question. She would come by in a couple of hours to examine me, and we would call her if we needed her to come earlier. I felt a bit like a kid playing hooky from school. I got to stay home from work ... hooray!

I went into the kitchen and started to prepare some raspberry leaf tea. Might as well be prepared, I thought. I sent a few e-mails, still having contractions every five minutes. It was during one of these that I noticed an odd sensation of liquid trickling out of me.

My first thought was, "Oh, God, I'm peeing myself now! What on earth is up with that?" My second thought was, "Oh, gosh, what if it's not pee? What if I'm bleeding?"

I rushed to the washroom to investigate and breathed a sigh of relief that the liquid was not blood. It was colorless, but I noted a funny but familiar odor: it smelled like semen, not what I'd expected. I didn't know what this meant, but I figured that it warranted a call to Fariba just to check in.

When I mentioned that I had some liquid coming out with the contractions, the first question she asked was this: "Does it smell like semen?" "Umm, yes," I replied, while thinking, "Oh, lovely, I'm the girl who knows what semen smells like!" Her voice reflected clearly that things had changed. "That is amniotic fluid. Your water has broken; you will be having your baby today!" Today. Today!

As I had tested positive for group B streptococcus (GBS) a few weeks earlier, Fariba asked that I remain lying down as a safety precaution for the baby until she could arrive and ensure that the fluid was clear. When she arrived at our home at nine o'clock that morning, she did a brief check and found that I was one centimeter dilated and seventy percent effaced. I had no idea at the time what effaced meant, but I thought it sounded pretty good to already be at seventy. My water had partially broken, and Fariba explained that meant there was a tear somewhere in the sac, but the fluid was clear, so there was no need to be concerned for the baby. I was given my first intravenous drip of antibiotics (because I had tested positive for strep), then she left to attend some of her appointments with other clients.

Darren and I were ecstatic: our baby was coming! We had gone shopping the previous afternoon and bought loads of fresh fruit and juices, and we spent the next little while preparing wonderful fruit bowls to eat throughout the day. I didn't have an appetite, but I think that had more to do with my excitement than anything caused by labor. I nibbled on cherries and sipped peach-grape juice through contractions that were still pretty mild.

From time to time, I'd have a contraction that would take my breath away. Afterward I'd say to Darren, "Oooooh, that was a big one!" having no idea at that time what big would come to mean. We spent the morning inflating the birth ball and sorting through the teeny little outfits that we'd bought for our baby, choosing the one that we wanted for the birth. We laughed and chattered on, nibbling on fruit and drinking water and juice. It was exciting but in a very relaxed kind of way.

As the afternoon approached, the intensity of my contractions began to build a bit. I found that I didn't want to continue talking through them as I had before, and it was often necessary to stop in my tracks and lean up against the wall for support. Darren was incredible. At the first sign that a contraction was coming, he'd be by my side in a split second; he applied counterpressure to my lower back and spoke softly to me, telling me just how wonderfully I was doing. As the flow of the contraction washed over me, I'd hear his voice strong and clear, and it gave me strength. His belief in me was contagious: I believed in me too.

Fariba returned just after two o'clock that afternoon. Since the contractions had become so much stronger in the past hour or two, I was eager to hear how much I was dilated. Five centimeters? Maybe seven? Nope...three. To say that I wasn't a bit discouraged would be dishonest. I felt my shoulders slump ever so slightly, but Fariba remained ever positive.

"You are progressing so well!" she said. "This baby will be here even sooner than I first thought!" Hearing those words bolstered my spirits more than anyone can ever know. To hear not only that everything was going well, but also that it was going even more quickly than she'd expected renewed my energy levels.

My memories of that afternoon are a bit hazy compared with earlier in the day. As labor progressed, I was completely and intently focused on the ebb and release of each contraction so that time faded out and became fuzzy and dream-like. I remember that I kept moving as much as was possible for me. I tried laboring on the birth ball for a time but discovered that my contractions seemed to die down when I was using it. This was something that I did not want! My instincts told me that keeping my labor active would be the best thing I could do for our baby. I wasn't necessarily trying to speed up the process of labor, but I didn't want to do anything that would get in its way.

I remember sitting on the toilet quite a lot, not to use the bathroom, but I discovered that the position made my contractions more intense and more frequent. It just felt right to me.

Toward late afternoon Darren and I decided to try a walk around the block. As we stepped outside, I was able to take in the kind of day my baby would be born into: muggy with a bit of rain beginning to fall, and refreshingly cool air. I noticed just how quiet everything was. I don't remember a single car driving along the road, and the air was still; not a noise broke the silence.

Walking itself proved to be a bit more to handle than I had expected. The contractions were much more intense now, and I soon realized how wonderful it was to have a strong wall to lean against. When I felt the approaching wave of a contraction, we'd stop and I would lean against Darren for its entirety. It took us almost a half hour to make what is normally a ten-minute walk around the block, and I was quite sure that would be my last little outdoor jaunt during this labor. Was I glad to return home!

Fariba had told us that she would return around six o'clock. I had a bit of a countdown going on for the last hour and a half before she came, which in hindsight, tells a lot about how intense my labor had become. Six o'clock came … and went. Somehow in my mind I thought her arrival would speed up the whole process; somehow her presence would make it all happen much faster. She arrived half an hour later, and I was sure that we'd be coming into the last stretch.

In truth, I was eighty-five percent effaced but just four centimeters dilated. Four! Just one centimeter gained through all those contractions? Over four hours and just one centimeter? I was bewildered. Surely I had come along farther than that. How could it be?

I began to envision a long night ahead of me. Fariba, seeing my discouraged posture, reassured me that everything was going very well and said that she would like to check my cervix on the next contraction. I could feel another building, a very strong one, and as it built up into its peak, Fariba exclaimed, "You are dilating now! You have just gone to six centimeters!"

I was rejuvenated. My body was doing what it knew how to do, and I once again felt fully confident that I could do this. I could do this!

I spent the next hour laboring in the bathtub. I know now that this was during the period of transition, and in my memory it was one of dizzying sensations and profound concentration. The water was cool, and I lay back against the slope of our tub with Darren sitting by my side and Fariba near my feet. It was complete. The whole of my mind and body was committed to the effort of creating a birthing canal for our baby, and I was very strongly aware of that.

Soon the contractions grew into pairs: one would reach its peak, begin the slightest retraction, only to meet with the rising of another. Honestly, my thoughts at this time were simple: "No fair!" I even laughed a little at myself. I wanted that delicious break between contractions, but at the same time I felt that this was good. It meant that we were coming nearer to our baby.

Just when I first began to think, "I don't know if I can do this anymore," Fariba told me that it was time to leave the bath; it was time to begin to push. I was fully dilated. This was it!

We returned to the living room, where we had prepared an area for birthing. Fariba showed me how to lie inclined on the couch, bringing my knees up close to my chest. She told me to try to push with the next contraction. I felt a most incredible urge to push, and it was amazing how the sensation of pain I'd felt during contractions seemed to be all but gone now. I pushed with every bit of strength I could muster. I don't know what I had expected, exactly—nothing specific—but this was hard. A couple more contractions came, and with each I pushed, Fariba's quiet and calm voice guiding and assuring me.

Right around that time Bridgett, our backup midwife, arrived. I heard Darren letting her in, and she breezed into the living room with a confident air of "let's get to it" efficiency. It's kind of amusing, actually, meeting someone for the first time when your knees are up around your shoulders and your bottom is kissing the sky, not necessarily one of my most dignified moments.

Even though I was a bit preoccupied, I remember seeing Bridgett standing to one side as I entered into another contraction, head kind of tilted to the side and frowning slightly as she puzzled over something. No sooner had the contraction ended than she said, "Fariba, that position just isn't doing anything for her. Let's try something else."

She strode across the room (okay, if it requires only two steps, is it still considered striding?) and put a hand on my shoulder. "I'd like you to come down onto the floor. Yup, that's right: onto your knees and supporting your upper body on the couch." Someone had placed a couch cushion onto the floor, quickly covered in a black garbage bag and pillow case, and I eased myself down into place just as another contraction began to swell inside me.

Wow! What a difference this change in position made! This time, as the contraction peaked I felt a whole new strength behind my pushing, and I could begin to feel the baby moving outward in the birth canal. This was really going to happen and pretty darn soon.

I wish that I could pay proper tribute to the actual birthing of Tessa, but the truth is that my memory of that time is hazy. For one thing, even though I pushed for forty-five minutes, it felt like only five or ten. Where the rest of that half hour went is beyond me.

What I most remember is feeling very focused during my contractions. It was almost rhythmic, and although this sounds silly, I'd describe it as rather painless, painless but exhausting, more exhausting than anything I've ever done in my life, any mountain climb, any run—infinitely more. I'd push and push through the contractions, then collapse onto the couch with my face flat on the cushion. I learned that by holding tight with my vaginal muscles between contractions, I could keep the baby from receding back into the canal. It was the strangest combination of being almost comatose yet still completely aware. It's as close to an out-of-body experience as I have ever experienced.

I remember Fariba telling me to reach in and feel how close our baby was. I did, and it was the most incredible thing, this crinkly little head that didn't feel much like a head at all. Cool stuff. Darren was at my side, and I could hear his voice talking softly to me, telling me how well I was doing and how close we were to holding our baby.

Before I knew it, Fariba was telling me that on my next contraction she wanted me to come to an upright position on one foot and one knee. Darren and I were about to catch our baby, our own baby! I was awestruck. Silently I came up, and before I even had a chance to think "This is it!" the contraction came, and I felt a most intense burn as our baby's head emerged, a burning like I'd never yet experienced but not truly painful.

Instantly I felt a wet, warm, and a more than slightly slippery baby! Darren helped me catch our baby in both of his hands, and together we cradled this little person, the first hands to welcome our babe into the world. I have no idea how long we stayed in this moment. In some ways it feels like it was a lifetime.

After a moment of wonder, quietly greeting our new little one, Darren asked, "Do we have a boy or a girl?" to which Fariba laughed and said, "Well, look for yourself." So we did. It was a girl. I was so surprised. For most of the pregnancy I had believed that I would have a boy. I was delighted and overcome with emotion. A daughter. My own little girl.

She was beautiful, raven-black hair damp against her head, a small, crinkled face, and oh, so tiny. She was amazingly quiet, looking around with such alert eyes but hardly making a sound. And so pink! Pink and naked and perfect.

While I expelled the placenta (which, incidentally, took a whole lot longer than I had ever imagined), Bridgett had Tessa behind me, gently blowing oxygen over her face. "She's perfect," Bridgett explained, "I just need her to flail for me. She's just so calm!" It felt like forever to me, far too long to be away from my girl, even though it probably took only a few minutes. She must have become tired from the wait too, and she let out a little squawk, waving her arms and legs in protest. Good girl!

By that time I'd delivered the placenta and eagerly gathered her up into my arms again. (Gosh, she was tiny!) We retreated to the softly lit bedroom to lie together, our first cuddle in the outside world. Bridgett came along to help me with our first breastfeeding, showing me how to brush my nipple across my girl's mouth to encourage her to "latch on." Well, let's just say that we both gave it our best go and that it was a good bit more challenging than either of us had probably imagined. But just holding her, my Tessa, feeling her suckle blindly against my breast, hearing her little sighs and snorts was simply amazing.

Two hours passed in the blink of an eye. Our midwives, bless their hearts, left the three of us to ourselves, cleaning up as much as they could while we enjoyed our togetherness. I wish I could somehow recall what little whispers we shared with Tessa, though maybe it is best that they remain somewhere deep in our unconscious memories. No doubt, those first murmurings, filled with love and breathless exhilaration, can somehow never be recaptured.

Fifteen hours, from start to finish. While I don't know if I'd go so far as to say that I wish it had taken longer (transition is no fun), in a way I feel like I would have liked for it to have gone on forever. It was painful, but somehow this also intensified the joy that I felt. Looking back, it is the joy that I remember best. Perhaps this is Mother Nature's way of keeping these babies coming. If so, she's darn clever!

◯

COLETTE STOEBER'S BIRTH STORY

THIS IS A sad story. But there is good in it: strength, courage, and hope. So I will write it.

I will open with a snapshot: September seventh at one minute past midnight. I am lying on a bed in a hospital room. To my left is my husband, Michael; to my right is my mother; and near the foot of the bed is my midwife, Susan. The rest of the room is filled with a vast array of nameless and, as far as I am concerned, faceless physicians and nurses. My daughter, Catherine Anne, has just been born.

We hadn't intended to have such a crowd at the birth of our first child. The event we had planned was much more intimate: just us and our midwives. The medical team became necessary, however, when we discovered on my due date—nearly three weeks earlier—that Catherine had a chromosomal abnormality: trisomy 18.

Her chances of living with such a condition were negligible. Few trisomy 18 babies are carried to term, and of those that are, few survive childbirth. The long-term prognosis is, in the words of one of the many physicians we spoke to during those seemingly endless three weeks, "very, very poor." Most babies will not live longer than two days. And, indeed, Catherine died exactly thirty-six hours after she was born.

That is the sad part: that we lost our daughter, that our midwife found herself attending the funeral of the baby she expected to usher into life, that we faced a terrible time of grieving.

As Michael and I began our bereavement counseling, it slowly became clear that our story of loss was different from others. Most parents who had faced circumstances similar to ours seemed to be experiencing much more shock, isolation, and unresolved anger. When we looked back on Catherine's birth and death, we began to see that all of the choices and decisions we had made throughout my pregnancy, choices made in the expectation of a normal baby, had led us to a place of great strength, a place where we were the ones in control, the ones who owned the process. When we were suddenly faced with such a grim reality, we had the confidence to ask many questions and make our own decisions. And we had a powerful support system in place.

From the beginning of my pregnancy, we chose a natural path toward childbirth. We decided on little or no testing. In my birth plan I envisioned no medical or drug intervention. I had friends and family who had had very positive experiences with and were strong proponents of midwives, so I was familiar with the philosophies and practices. I absolutely wanted to be in the care of a midwife.

The advantages of a midwife-managed birth are so clear, in fact, that I am constantly amazed that any woman would choose anything else. Susan was on call for us twenty-four hours a day from the moment we entered her care, for the nearly forty-one weeks of my pregnancy. Our monthly checkups routinely ran over an hour. We were fully informed of all medical issues, and we had complete and immediate access to the treatments and tests available. She left the decision making up to us and supported our choices. Further, she treated the baby with growing affection. I remember in particular her own pleasure at the first sound of the heartbeat. By the end of the pregnancy she knew us and our baby in a way that no physician could have.

An ultrasound in the first trimester would probably have indicated Catherine's chromosomal abnormality. This was the medical world's recurring question, asked in gently accusing tones, after our very late discovery: why didn't you test earlier? Because termination was not an option for us, Michael and I had decided against doing any testing, avoiding even ultrasounds. In spite of this, we did submit to a very late ultrasound at thirty-two weeks on Susan's advice, because of low fundal height measurements.

At that time, the baby was merely noted to be small (in the twenty-sixth percentile), and no anomalies were seen. The irony of course is that in the end it was our continued ignorance of Catherine's nature that allowed us to completely invest in and enjoy her life, the only life she was capable of living. Early testing and discovery would simply have resulted in our immediate grief and anguished doubts over terminating the pregnancy. As it is, she lived out her natural life from start to finish. Her true nature was not revealed to us until the precise day she was due to emerge into the world.

Susan scheduled the second ultrasound on my due date because the small fundal measurements persisted in the last month of pregnancy; she wanted us to proceed into overdue time with confidence. On August nineteenth, I found myself lying on my back, thirty-eight weeks pregnant, on a cold table in a curtained-off cubicle.

Michael was in the waiting room, not allowed to come in because of the cramped space. As I lay there, becoming more and more uncomfortable, I watched the demeanor of the ultrasound technician shift from a relaxed, routine friendliness to grim silence. The examination went on and on; it was clear that something was very wrong. By the time I emerged from the room, I was shaking. I felt I had entered another world: the world of after.

They had discovered a heart defect, brain stem anomalies, an abnormality in the kidney, overlapping of the fingers with clenched hands, and an excess of amniotic fluid. All combined to indicate a serious but undetermined chromosomal abnormality. We weren't told any of these details at the lab, of course. We were told to go immediately to our midwife's office.

We rushed into Susan's office and found her holding the faxed report in her hands. She had already put in a call to a genetic counselor at the prenatal diagnosis unit of our local hospital, and she began to break the news to us of the serious implications of the findings. At this point they couldn't be clear on the exact nature of the condition, but the sheer number of abnormalities discovered indicated something very serious: either trisomy 13 or 18. Our baby would be, at the very best, seriously disabled, physically and neurologically.

As we sat there stunned, Susan gently began the onerous process of setting up and transferring our care into the appropriate medical hands: specialists, obstetricians, geneticists, and neonatalists at two local hospitals, where they eventually determined through an amniocentesis that the baby was trisomy 18.

We received excellent care at these hospitals. The physicians were thorough, informative, and patient, answering our many questions with a sympathetic and respectful professionalism. But Susan remained our principal caregiver as the pregnancy dragged on. In spite of our changed circumstances, we wanted to make Catherine's birth as close to our original plan as we could. Although our obstetrician offered to medically induce labor, we decided to wait for it to begin naturally. Susan remained on call to us. She helped me to encourage labor through herbal and homeopathic methods and through cervical stretching. When I finally went into labor, she remained at home with us for the first stages, took us to the hospital when it was time, and remained to coach me through delivery.

Catherine was born with a minimum of fuss. I arrived at the hospital almost fully dilated so that as soon as they got me settled on the bed, I was ready to begin pushing. The obstetrician on call was very busy that night and kept leaving the room between contractions. The triangle of Michael, my mom, and Susan kept me anchored and focused. The labor, which lasted six hours in total, ended with less than fifteen minutes of pushing. By the time Catherine arrived, crying with a sudden, brief burst of energy that shocked everyone in the room, the neonatal physicians had arrived to take over her care.

Susan was the one who finally broke the physician's silence to tell me it was a girl. She was the one who took Catherine from the hands of the neonatalist, laid her on my chest and tried, with me, to coax her to nurse. She conferred with the medical staff, arranged a private room for us, and spoke with family members who were waiting for news. She stayed with us at the hospital until late into that night, then returned the next night to sit and listen with us to our baby's determined breathing. Even as I write this, I am overwhelmed by the vivid memory of the three of us sitting silent in the dim room, the sound of Catherine's dogged, rasping breath filling the spaces between us.

Later she showed me how to bind my breasts with cabbage leaves to stop my milk, Catherine's milk, from coming in. Finally, she was there to grieve with us at Catherine's funeral.

I will end this sad story with another snapshot, the part of this story that is about hope: December first, one year later, at one minute past one in the morning. I am in a hospital room. To my left is Michael, to my right is my mother, and at the foot of the bed is Susan. The only other people in the room are the backup midwife and the midwife in training.

My daughter Charlotte Clare has just been born and her cries fill the air of the room. Charlotte came into the world with both of her arms stretched upward above her head, reaching for life, diving into life, which she continues to do every day.

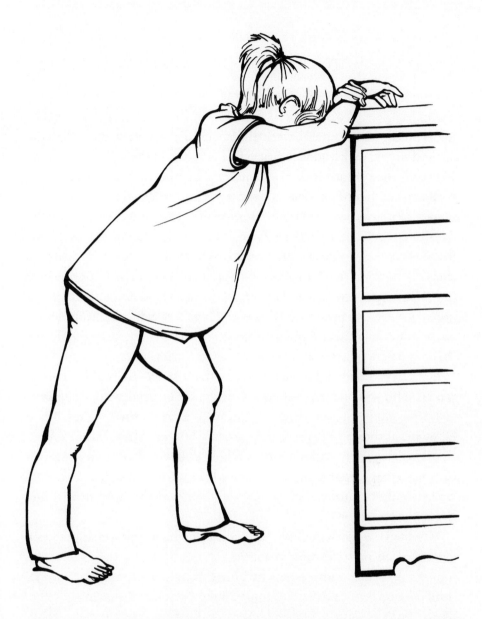

FORWARD-LEANING POSITIONS, especially when sitting with the legs open or standing up with one leg forward, allow for an optimal alignment of baby, uterus, and hips. The force of gravity is an added bonus because it is pointed in the same direction as the focus of the contractions and the exit point of the baby, the cervix. The standing position with one leg forward and bent in a slight lunge opens up the pelvis while at the same time nudging the baby toward the cervix. The expansion of the pelvis can make the difference in birthing large babies or babies in less than optimal positions. When one position no longer seems to be helping a woman cope with contractions, she should be free to try another. If she is too tired to move, her labor support people should be there to help her.

JODY FRANCIS'S BIRTH STORY

MY HUSBAND GORD and I were thrilled to find out we were pregnant (the hallmark emotion with a planned pregnancy). I immediately began talking to my three sisters, who had already had a combined total of twelve babies, to get a recommendation for a good physician. Of the twelve babies, eleven had been born in hospitals with physicians and one was born at home. My sister Kim had had five caesarean sections, the first deemed an emergency due to failure to progress and the next four scheduled because no physician thought she should try a vaginal birth after caesarean (VBAC). When she became pregnant with her sixth baby, she read the book *Silent Knife: Vaginal Birth after Cesarean and Cesarean Prevention* by Nancy Wainer Cohen and Lois Estner and began attending VBAC meetings. She became convinced that her caesarean sections hadn't been necessary and that she probably could successfully deliver a baby vaginally.

Kim proceeded to hire a midwife and, with the support of her obstetrician, was planning a vaginal birth after caesarean at the hospital, with the midwife providing labor support. As things turned out, when she was in labor at home and at the point of needing to go to the hospital, she told the midwife she didn't want to go and the baby was born at home. Besides creating a bit of a mess to clean up since it wasn't planned, the birth went well and Kim and her husband were thrilled. She had vaginally delivered a healthy baby girl after five caesarean sections.

My initial reaction was, "They were so lucky nothing went wrong." As I soon discovered, my attitude would change.

Just weeks after Kim's experience, my other sister Leanne had had her third hospital birth and was still complaining about the episiotomy from her second birth, about the negative effects of the drugs she was given, about delivering her baby while on her back, about the physician barely making it to the hospital before the baby was born, and on and on.

Based on both of my sisters' most recent birth experiences, Gord and I decided to meet with the midwife and see if she was qualified and competent. I suspected that I might have a long labor like my sister Kim, and I didn't want an unnecessary caesarean. I called the midwife, Donna, and made an appointment with her.

Donna came to our apartment on a Saturday afternoon, and we talked for over an hour. Gord and I were very impressed with her knowledge, professionalism, and warmth. We were excited to work with her over the course of the pregnancy and birth. We had total confidence in her background, experience, and expertise. We trusted her to assist us in having a wonderful, safe birth, at home, we hoped.

The pregnancy went well. I saw both Donna and a recommended physician throughout. Both monitored me in exactly the same way: measuring, weighing, taking blood tests and urine tests, and checking blood pressure, though I found that visits at the midwife's office were somehow friendlier and more relaxed. My blood pressure was creeping up throughout the pregnancy, and there was concern that if it continued to climb, I would need to have the baby at the hospital, which I didn't want to do.

To help lower my blood pressure, I left work a few weeks before my due date to relax at home. It seemed to work. Or was it the garlic capsules I was taking that were also helping?

Tuesday morning, just a few days before my due date, I lost the mucus plug. I was so excited that I had to call my sisters to let them know that labor would probably start soon. Sure enough, after lunch my contractions officially began to arrive, about every ten minutes and lasting for thirty seconds.

I must be built like my sister Kim because my labor progressed very slowly. Gord had called Donna right away; she told us to call her back when we needed her. Just before midnight he called her again to let her know that contractions were coming about every four to five minutes and lasting about forty seconds. Donna arrived shortly afterward.

This continued throughout the night. By five in the morning, I was dilated to four centimeters and the contractions were two minutes apart, lasting about fifty seconds each.

My poor, sweet husband was awake all night with me, writing down every contraction and how long it lasted (at my request, since he would have much rather been sleeping). Because I was progressing slowly, Donna returned home for a few hours, instructing us to call again when contractions became longer.

By noon on Wednesday, twenty-four hours after contractions had begun, they were lasting a minute or longer and coming every three or four minutes. Just before three in the afternoon, my water broke while I was lying on my side in bed. Fortunately we were prepared. Gord called Donna, and from then on contractions continued to get stronger. There was some meconium staining in the water but not enough to concern the midwife, so I was able to remain at home. My blood pressure was "behaving," and the baby was doing well during the contractions.

By six in the evening, Donna had called for Noreen, the backup midwife, to come since the birth was close. I spent a lot of time alternating between leaning over my bed, sitting on the toilet, and sitting on the birthing stool. I reached ten centimeters by eight forty-five PM, and after I pushed for fifty minutes while squatting on the birthing stool, our beautiful daughter was born after thirty-two hours of labor.

She was immediately placed on my bare chest and wrapped in a warm towel. What an amazing experience to push a baby out! She was beautiful and had long skinny feet.

Fifteen minutes later I delivered the placenta. There was no tearing, just serious bruising, so no stitches were required.

We were so happy and excited. I climbed back into my bed, freshly made with warm flannel sheets, while she was weighed and measured in front of me. I was again holding our gorgeous baby and began breastfeeding her. What a funny thought that all of a sudden my breasts had food for a baby in them!

It was soon time to phone the proud grandparents to give them the exciting news: Zoë Lynn was seven pounds eight ounces and was twenty-one inches long. She was perfect!

I am convinced that had I delivered in a hospital, my birth experience would have been considerably different, probably much more negative and dramatic because I did progress so slowly. I don't believe most physicians would have been able to sit back and watch; most would have been putting me on an intravenous drip or breaking my water, which would probably have led to more interventions, including an epidural, drugs, an episiotomy, forceps, or caesarean, none of which I wanted.

I was never worried about the length of my labor since the midwives were monitoring the baby and me throughout and provided so much support and encouragement. And it was so nice being at home in my own environment!

Birth experienced the way I experienced it is so amazingly empowering, such a wonderful, satisfying experience. I can only wish that all women could experience birth in such a positive way. Labor in childbirth is hard work but is most definitely worth it!

Reinekke Lengelle's birth story

I LIKE TO call myself "spiritual" as opposed to religious. Expressions like "judge not and you shall not be judged" usually seem a little severe to me, but that changed when I had my daughter Sophia and went from being a brow-beating natural childbirth advocate to a damned epidural recipient. I am still very much an advocate of natural birth, only now I've developed some compassion for myself and for those who have less than idyllic birth experiences.

Let me tell you about my seventy-hour tale. I went into labor on a Wednesday evening. It was October first, and I was glad to see the show of bloody mucus that heralded the arrival of our first child. I was already two weeks overdue and was eager for the birth process to begin. My husband Keath and I felt wonderfully prepared and my pregnancy had gone extremely well, aside from a lot of nausea in the first trimester. We had also had an in-depth, loving education from our midwife and were ready for a home birth.

I slept for about five hours that Wednesday night and woke up Thursday to heavier contractions. Most of the day, the contractions seemed to get stronger and stronger, though they were a bit irregular. We decided to call Susan, our midwife, and keep her posted, but didn't have her come until Friday morning at eight o'clock. Then things seemed to get under way fairly well, and I had dilated about four centimeters by three o'clock that afternoon. I started to have some back pain, and Keath and I went for a walk around the neighborhood, stopping every so often so I could lean on a tree and breathe through another contraction. It was a beautiful autumn day.

By evening the pain was predictably becoming harder to bear. My mom and Keath took turns rubbing my back. Later they helped Susan set up the big birthing pool in the kitchen where the sun shone through the patio doors and reflected on the water. I could breathe well through the contractions but the back pain was getting worse. At one point I got out of the birthing pool for a while and started crawling around the living room and hallway. That evening sometime around eight o'clock, Susan informed me that I was about seven centimeters dilated and, in hopes of getting things under way a little better, I agreed to have her break my water.

The irregular contractions went on well into the night, and I tried to vent the pain from the back labor by moaning deeply. I sat on the toilet for a while, and it almost seemed like my body wanted to show me a push but couldn't get it to really happen. Though at this point I was still willing to appreciate all of the pain as part of the job, I found that by the early hours of the morning I became very discouraged—finding I had not made any progress with dilation. By about three AM, my mother and the midwife started to drop off to sleep, and that did not boost my morale or confidence, either. With my labor stalled, I decided I wanted to go to the hospital and see if a change of scene and some artificial pain relief would help.

Once there, I was checked again and medical staff confirmed I was still only seven to eight centimeters dilated, stuck just before "transition," the hardest and most painful part of labor before the pushing stage. The nurse on duty helped me get comfortable under the hot shower and administered morphine, the second sign of failure (the first was going to the hospital at all). I became drowsy, but the pain didn't feel like it had really diminished. I fell asleep between each contraction.

The obstetrician came in and informed me that my baby was posterior (the baby's spine lined up with my spine instead of the other way around). This was probably the reason I was experiencing heavy back labor and probably why my cervix wasn't opening very well: the baby's head wasn't pushing down on it in a way that helped open me up. I felt a bit better at having the "diagnosis" and disappointed in the midwife that she hadn't thought to suggest that this might have been what was keeping my labor from progressing. In hindsight, and with more knowledge of the physiology of birth, I realize that my own performance angst may have played a substantial role in the long struggle as well.

The sun was just rising on Saturday, October fourth, when Keath and I walked through the halls of the hospital wondering what we should do now that not only our bodies but our options seemed exhausted. I was stumped and afraid and still did not want an epidural, not only because it felt like the ultimate failure and unnatural way to birth, but also because I feared that the epidural might actually paralyze me. Keath felt at an impasse too. Indirectly I was presenting him with a kind of ultimate dilemma, which went something like this: I can see my wife die of pain and heaven knows when this baby will be born or I can see her choose the epidural that she doesn't want and fears.

We came back to the labor room still not knowing what to do. I remember lying in the dark for a while and turning to the nurse (Laurie was her name) and saying something like "I feel terrible." She took my hand and in the sweetest voice she said, "Oh, but you're doing so well." And she really meant it. I was so grateful to her!

By the afternoon (some threats of a caesarean had already been uttered) the anesthesiologist came in to offer me an epidural. I asked him: "What are my chances of getting paralyzed?" He replied: "What are the chances that you're going to fall out of this bed?" Though it sounded rather unprofessional, his answer was strangely comforting.

I have to mention that during the entire labor I never once worried about the baby but had a solid sense that "she" was fine. Keath stayed with me, my mother was still with us, and Susan and the hospital staff were working together in way that was more than civil. (Note that without hospital privileges, Susan had lost her role as my primary caregiver.)

Saying "yes" to the epidural was quite possibly the most difficult decision I had ever made. The right half of my body felt completely dead (my leg lay like a log that didn't belong to me) and although my left side still pulsed with blunted contractions, I was able to sleep for a few hours. Soon I was completely dilated and felt the faint urge to push. By about six PM I started pushing with the help of the monitor that showed the contractions because I had only a vague awareness of them.

A nurse spurred me like a football coach, and because I couldn't feel the contractions well enough to trust my body, her prompting was helpful. There were still threats uttered about giving me an episiotomy, but I spoke up clearly and said that was absolutely not going to happen. I had done my research on this intervention and found that often a natural tear is preferable to a deep cut that takes weeks to heal, especially since many birthing women suffer no damage to the perineum at all. Saying "no" to this procedure also allowed me to salvage at least a shred of my hope to have a natural birth.

The epidural wore off in time for me to feel the pushing contractions that finally led to the painful crowning and the birth of our daughter Sophia Aurora at two minutes past eight that Saturday evening, October fourth.

Wow! Here she was, so healthy and alert! Our beautiful baby girl. We had done it. We had done it with the help of a midwife, my husband, my mother, the hospital staff, morphine, an epidural, and my deep determination to have the most natural birth possible. It may not sound so natural to some, but I did come out of it without an episiotomy, caesarean section, or forceps/suction delivery. And in a strange way, I had the birth my way the whole highway: each decision was truly mine in the end.

I've argued that if I had been less anxious or had held views about childbirth that were less adamant, I might have had an easier birth, or at the very least been less disappointed with the way it unfolded. Even knowing Sophia was posterior or that the "latent" phase of labor can actually drag on for days, I suppose, might have given me reason to relax and cope for a longer time without drugs. And yet, listing the what-ifs doesn't fully acknowledge that this was simply the birth I had; no amount of reflection can change the facts. The gift that has been *born* from this experience is not only a beautiful daughter but a changed me: I am no longer a brow-beating natural-birth advocate (full of judgments) but a woman who is invested in supporting other women who want a natural birth whatever the outcome (releasing judgments). With that in heart and mind, I'll finish my story with a poem for you and me:

> So forgive yourself,
> for not being perfect.
> For saying, enough is enough.
> For setting out a dream
> and then landing on the bed of nails.
> So forgive yourself,
> and don't say "I didn't do it right,"
> because you did.
> So forgive yourself,
> for being the judge
> of your own heart.

GUDRUN VON SELZAM'S BIRTH STORY

ON SPRING EQUINOX day, our daughter Robin's second birthday, we found out that we were pregnant. How exciting! I knew exactly when it had happened, a very special, loving, beautiful, romantic evening, and I remember thinking it would be the perfect time for some little soul to choose us. As we found out twenty weeks later, not for just one little soul. After an intuitive feeling I decided to have an ultrasound, and sure enough there they were: two babies, perfectly developed, the left one head down, the right one in breech position. We were thrilled! So was every one of our friends, family, and our midwives, who were comfortable with our plan to have a home birth.

I loved being pregnant and having these little miracles growing inside me. Three souls, three heart beats, three in one body was fascinating!

In the next few months I started reading about twin births, but all the books I found, except one, Elizabeth Noble's *Having Twins,* stressed the complications, the danger, the high rate of caesareans, and the fact that most twin babies come early, are too small, and so on. They all focused on what could go wrong, so I stopped reading anything else and concentrated on the positive attitude in Noble's book.

I started picturing myself in our beautiful sunroom, in the birthing pool, having around six hours of labor followed by a wonderful water birth, then getting out of the tub and birthing the second baby soon after. I picked a due date in my fortieth week, November twenty-second, a new moon and cusp day of Scorpio, my partner Ted's zodiac sign, and told everyone that I would have the babies on that day, preferably in the afternoon.

As my due date was getting closer and closer, I was amazed by how easily everything was going. I had expected to feel at least some discomfort—feeling too heavy, getting back pains, or something—but there was hardly anything to complain about at all.

On the twenty-second, we were ready. I felt so prepared for having our babies that day (in the afternoon, remember?). We had done a sweet-grass ceremony, the house was unusually clean and tidy, our birth supplies—essential oils, some good music, Bach flower remedies, candles, cushions, towels, and the birth bag from the midwives—were in place, the champagne was in the fridge, even the lasagna to feed the midwives was thawed! And my chosen due date passed without event.

So I learned my lesson: Our babies have their own minds and will come when they are ready, not when I want them to. I was fine with that. Maybe the house was too clean for them.

Thirty-six hours later, on November twenty-fourth at one in the morning—clocks can become meditation objects when you are starting labor—I woke up with a mild contraction. It was definitely not a Braxton Hicks, so I went to the bathroom to check for more exciting signs, and there was the pink show and the diarrhea.

I woke Ted, and we timed the contractions: they were ten minutes apart and around one minute long. At one thirty AM, we phoned our friend Teri, support person for our daughter, and Barbara, our midwife, who told us to call her back whenever labor picked up or we wanted her to come. Okay.

I went to the bathroom again and was hit by a huge, powerful, strong, long contraction that nearly threw me off the toilet. I remember pushing my hands against the wall in front of me as hard as I could. There it was: I suddenly knew once again how it felt to be in labor. How could I have forgotten?

After I had another contraction like that one, I told Ted to call Barbara back. Yes, a hot bath was a good idea. Contractions hit me hard, but I felt quite under control. I was sitting in my bathtub in our tiny bathroom picturing this huge wave and my going with it. After the peak of each contraction I would slowly roll off the wave. This worked great for the time being.

Teri and Barbara arrived, then Robin woke up. Barbara brought the birthing pool but didn't have the electric pump, so she phoned our second midwife, Noreen, for it and invited the other two midwives, Wendy and Kerstin, to come.

I suddenly got this very clear feeling that there was no way we would get the pool ready in time. Just about when Kerstin and Noreen arrived, at around three twenty-five AM, I had to change my position from sitting to hands and knees and got this irresistible urge to push. So I did, trusting my body, not listening to my brain that was telling me it must be far too early to push. (We hadn't done any checking.) I couldn't help it anyway.

It was a long, hard, powerful, loud push that brought the baby down to just an inch from being born. Wow!

Then a break ... greeting the midwives, laughing, talking, no pain at all.

Another long, hard, powerful, very loud push like an explosion, like thunder and lightning at the same time, and I pushed the baby out at once.

I just couldn't believe it: three thirty AM. It had been so fast, so intense, so perfect! In my arms I was holding a screaming, large, pink boy—and I had been convinced that this one was a girl. I sat down and held him, cleaned him, welcomed him, before Ted and Robin cut the cord and we got out of the water.

We went into the "birthing room," where the candles were still burning. I was happy to be in the middle of my birth experience, knowing that it would be just a short time until I could hold my second child, until everything would be over. I felt powerful and not one bit anxious about the second birth. Everything felt so right and good.

We were waiting for contractions to come back, and I was playing with that half empty belly of mine. I tried pushing without a contraction, which was very hard and did not seem to work well. Everyone seemed relaxed; there was no rush. Wendy arrived. All in the room seemed to find their way of being involved in the birth, and everyone was amazing. Ted was holding Benjamin Finn, our new son, who was snuggled into a warm towel; Kerstin filmed; Teri filmed or looked after Robin; Robin was on and off the bed, quietly observing, just being with me; Noreen was sitting on the birthing ball behind me, supporting my squatting or standing (what a job! I had all my weight on her); Wendy brought water, wiped my face with a cold washcloth, and gave me Rescue Remedy drops just when I needed them; Barbara did everything from checking where things were, to listening to the baby's heartbeat, to suggesting various positions, to giving me verbal support.

After we had tried all kinds of positions and the water bag just would not break, we decided to help it a bit. Then Barbara checked and felt little wiggling toes instead of the expected head. What a surprise! This was the "left" baby that had been head down on the first and only ultrasound. We all laughed and joked about the second ultrasound we had not done and were happy that we hadn't.

Then everything went very fast. One push got the little feet out. I touched them, thinking how tiny they were. Then one big great push and I birthed my baby, just like in the poem that hangs on my wall:

> ... an ancient river of blood
> will flow on through me,

when it comes time to see my child free;
just like a river that opens to the sea,
I am going to let my child flow right out of me ...

My second baby, Montana Geraldine, also said hello to this world with a loud scream. She seemed so petite, a beautiful, little, strong creature.

It was seven minutes after four in the morning. I still can't believe how quickly everything was over. Our family had grown from three to five in just three hours.

There I was, holding and nursing two perfect little babies in my arms, surrounded by loving, wonderful people and candlelight. I don't have the right words to describe these minutes, but they were incredible!

After the placenta was born—actually, there were two placentas grown together, a big one with a thick cord and a smaller one with a thinner cord— my babies and I took a relaxing warm bath.

Our next surprise came when they were weighed. Montana was six pounds three ounces and Benjamin was eight pounds, eleven ounces. I had carried almost fifteen pounds of babies.

The whole birth experience was amazing, but the most moving moment for me came afterward, a moment I'll never forget. It still brings tears to my eyes thinking of it. I needed some stitches, and every grown-up was busy holding babies, the lamp, my hand, or the needle. My intuitive little daughter Robin came onto the bed, sat right beside my head, and started singing for me: twinkle, twinkle, little star. . . . We sang and hummed together until everything was done. It was exactly what I needed at that time.

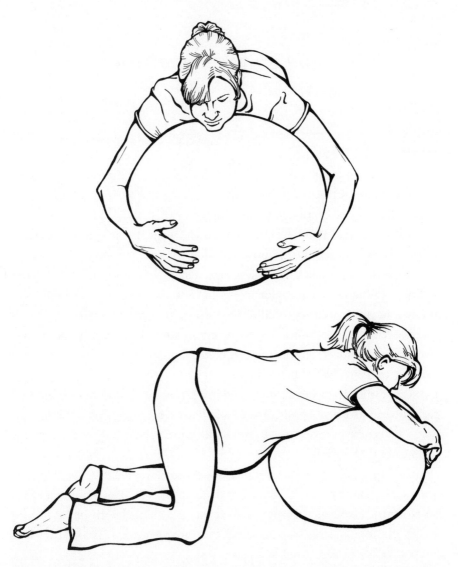

THE BIRTHING BALL is an amazing tool that adds comfort to pregnant women through-out pregnancy, labor, and birth. With it the woman can assume many supported positions in labor as her instincts dictate. A hospital birth can be made more comfortable by bring-ing a birthing ball since hospitals don't have many small and soft pieces of furniture, which women in labor are attracted to. In a home birth women can use their sofas, their pillows, their carpet, and their laundry baskets to lean over close to the ground. A birthing ball sat-isfies women's needs very well. The all-fours position with a birthing ball offers added sup-port and provides an excellent way to reduce stress on the lower back. A birthing ball is a common tool used in physical therapy, so it has many uses beyond pregnancy. A soft towel can be placed on the ball so that the woman's face can rest on it and not have to smell the plastic material or the dust on the ball.

Alyson Jones's birth story

NINE DAYS BEFORE my friend and I were supposed to board a plane to Thailand, I found out I was pregnant.

I was nineteen at the time, and this was an unexpected pregnancy. I saw a physician at the walk-in clinic and decided to continue with my plans to go to Asia. I felt it was early enough in my pregnancy that it would be okay to go.

I had always wanted to have children and had worked as a caregiver for years; however, I didn't feel very knowledgeable about pregnancy or childbirth. While I was away, I spent countless days and nights lying on beaches and trekking through jungles, exploring my life and the direction in which I was heading. At times I felt so afraid of the future that I contemplated staying in Asia forever. The apprehension of returning and telling my family and friends that I was pregnant was almost too much to consider.

After returning home, I found that my partner was now living with someone else. At first I was devastated; then my pregnancy hormones kicked in. I started to feel strong and positive and had a hard time feeling upset. While I was away, I had come to love the life growing inside me. Nothing could bring me down from that feeling.

I made an appointment to see my family doctor. I wanted to get tests done to make sure I hadn't picked up parasites while I was away. The night before my appointment I woke up because my bed was wet, stained with blood. Once I reached the toilet, a large blood clot dropped into the water. I crawled back into bed but couldn't sleep, sure I had miscarried.

In the morning I went to my appointment, feeling numb and emotionally spent. I had jet lag, and salmonella poisoning, as I learned later on, and thought I had just experienced a miscarriage. I hadn't; however, a major miscommunication occurred between my doctor and me, and I left his office still believing that I had miscarried. I trusted my doctor, and I did not doubt what he had said. I didn't ask for a pregnancy test, nor did he suggest one. That was the last time that I'll put that much trust in any health care provider.

Believing that I was no longer pregnant, I became deeply depressed. I couldn't stop thinking about how things would have been had I carried to term. It became necessary for me to get away, to leave my home town, so I moved to another city and stayed with a girlfriend.

A month went by. I drank, smoked, and took antibiotics to try to get rid of the bacteria I had acquired in Asia. I couldn't find work. I was throwing up every morning and felt nauseated all the time. I was at the end of my rope and trying to hold on.

Finally I went to see another doctor. She was nice, and I told her everything. She asked me if I thought I could still be pregnant. I answered her with a straightforward, "No!" I really didn't think there was any chance of that. We did a test. It was positive. I was four months pregnant.

I started to get nervous about all the horrible things I had done to my body and fetus in the past month and asked her if I could have done serious damage to my baby. She reassured me with words of wisdom that have stayed with me to this day. "Women who never drank or smoked and are very healthy sometimes have funny babies, and women who abuse and neglect their bodies can have perfectly healthy babies." I went for an ultrasound to make sure everything was all right, and she referred me to a maternity doctor who was accepting new patients.

I stayed where I was, and although I was living with my good friend and my mom had recently moved closer to me, I felt alone and alienated. I had lost my confidence and was scared. My new doctor was busy. I felt like I was rushed in and rushed out. I didn't have time to ask her questions. I felt like people looked at me like a naughty, single, pregnant woman. I know that a lot of those feelings were self-constructed, but that was how I felt.

I started volunteering at a children's recycled clothing store that happened to be run by four young single moms. These women were my goddesses, my breath, and my light. They quickly became close friends. As I spent more and more time at the store, I had the chance to hear stories about natural births and home births. I read the books lying around and asked many questions.

I did not feel fulfilled with the care I had been receiving from my doctor. It wasn't that she was mean; she just didn't seem to have time. She didn't care about who I was or what was important to me.

One day one of the women at the store suggested that I attend a midwives' information meeting. She had just had her second baby that week, at home, in her bathtub, with her family and midwives. She was radiant.

One night when I was at my mom's for dinner, we talked about midwives and home births. We talked about what we thought midwives did, and we both swore up and down that I would never consider a home birth.

That evening we attended an information meeting to learn more about available midwifery services. The meeting was amazing. The feeling in the room and the energy of the women was overpowering. The midwives showed videos and explained the role of a midwife. They answered our questions, and by the time the night was over, I knew who I wanted to attend my birth: Angela. We talked, bonding immediately. She checked her schedule for July and happily committed to being my midwife.

Things changed for me after that day. The difference in care was phenomenal! Angela's office was in an old Victorian-style house on a street lined with big, old trees. Inside, the walls were decorated with beautiful images of pregnant women and babies. There was a corkboard with pictures of recently delivered babies and a huge bookcase full of an amazing collection of books for borrowing.

At every appointment I was given the responsibility of weighing myself and peeing on a stick to check my pH balance. This may not seem like much, but when I went to my doctor to have an unfamiliar nurse weigh me on a big scale and ask me to pee in a jar, my self-confidence was taken away. When the nurse told me to undress and lie on the cold table in the tiny, stark room, I felt lonely and powerless. By showing me how to be in control of my own body and pregnancy, Angela helped me feel more powerful and confident than I had ever felt before.

During my appointments with Angela, which were usually an hour long, I never felt rushed and I asked all my questions. Angela also asked me questions about my past and what my plans were for my future. She informed me about the choices that I had regarding newborn tests and procedures. She never gave me her opinion. I believe that was one of the wisest things she did as a midwife. Angela knew the importance of a woman making her own choices and decisions.

As I got to know Angela and learned more about birthing, I decided to plan for a home birth. I felt no fear of staying at home to have my baby, and as my due date approached, I realized that I wasn't afraid of labor or birth. I wanted my birthing atmosphere to be dark, lit only by candles, with quiet music. With a home birth these options were open to me.

The day before my due date, I felt exhausted and crampy. I relaxed and played cribbage with my dad. Just before midnight, while I was struggling to fall asleep, my water broke. I was surprised; many people had told me that first babies were usually at least a week late. That was what I was expecting. I called my mom, who said she would be right over.

By the time she got to my apartment five minutes later, I was violently ill, throwing up and having diarrhea all at once, as well as contractions, which had come on fast. I was unable to communicate with my parents. My mom called Angela to check in, and she recommended that I try to get some rest, mentioning that the first stage could last awhile. Mom was wondering, "Whoa, if this lasts a long time, what will we do?"

For the next hour, my parents tried to talk to me and get some feedback as to how I was feeling and what stage I was in, but I was deep within myself and couldn't communicate with them. My dad thought at this point that my contractions were about two minutes apart and that we should call Angela again.

I had planned to have my baby at my aunt's house because my apartment was a small bachelor suite. My parents decided that it was time for us to go there. I refused. It was a difficult time for us all. Eventually my parents did convince me to get in the car, and we drove for fifteen minutes to get to my aunt's place. I will never drive during labor again. That was the hardest part of my entire labor. However, it was relaxing to arrive at the place where I had spent time preparing for my birth. Everything I wanted and needed was there.

As soon as I was settled, I felt the pressure of my baby pushing. I didn't understand how things were happening so fast. I hadn't learned about this in prenatal classes. It was now two forty-five in the morning. I told my mom I needed to push, and she called Angela, who said, "I'm on my way!"

Angela arrived at three fifteen AM, and I was very relieved to see her. She checked my dilation and let me know I was fully dilated. I was excited because I knew that my baby would soon be here. I was also elated that I could push and start the last stage of labor. For me, pushing was the best part of my labor because I could feel the progress my body was making and knew that the pain was a working pain.

I pushed for just under an hour. I stayed on my hands and knees until Angela whispered into my ear that my knees might hurt in the morning. She encouraged me to stand up and walk for a little while. Something about her words rang true, and I decided to get up and walk to the door. I made it halfway and stopped during a strong contraction. Gravity urged my baby's head to slip out, and with physical support from my dad and one more strong contraction, my nine-pound five-ounce healthy baby boy was born, after only four and a half hours of labor.

Leeum was born at 4:18 AM on July fifth. He was gorgeous. The atmosphere was perfect. My family and friends who were present made my birth experience the best possible transition to motherhood that I could have wished for.

Since then I have realized that my passion is to support women during their birthing experiences. I am now a doula, a breastfeeding counselor, and am working toward my ultimate goal of becoming a midwife.

The past four years of being a mother have been an incredible joy, and I am thankful every day for having such a wonderful son. My birth experience changed my life forever and inspired me to follow my heart's desires.

❧

KATIE SOKEY'S BIRTH STORY

IN MY MIND I had it all planned. Sarah, my oldest child, would arrive on Friday, which was Halloween. She and Zoe, my youngest, would go trick-or-treating together, and after that the baby would be born, November first maybe. Granted, Sarah would have to go right back when the weekend was over, but at least she would have been able to see the birth.

Of course I knew that it's silly to try to plan these things; a baby comes when it's ready. But, who knows? It could very well happen that way. My due date was November fourth, give or take a few days, and Zoe had been born a few days early. Why not this one?

Sarah is twelve years old. Unfortunately, because of a bad custody arrangement, she lives far away much of the time. Zoe is seven, and she and Sarah are great sisters and friends, despite being five years and often many miles apart from one another. Both Sarah and Zoe were born at home; both were amazing experiences that went extremely well. Feeling fortunate and grateful to have had two wonderful births, I wondered: could I be so lucky a third time?

This would be our last child, and my husband Michael wanted to know: girl or boy? So early on I had my first ever ultrasound. It showed a girl. Sarah and Zoe were thrilled; Michael braced himself for a lifetime of estrogen overload.

Well, Halloween came and went. So did my due date. I wasn't worried, though; I trusted my body to do what it knew how to do when it was time.

But the days kept going by, and the tension in our home grew. Zoe's outlet seemed to be picking fights with Grandma, who had arrived on November second to help with the baby, the baby who still hadn't arrived after a week. Then two weeks. Whenever I called Michael at work, he'd think I was in labor; finally, he told me not to call anymore unless I was. I awoke each day surprised to find that another night had passed and still no baby.

Even Shelly was becoming concerned. As a licensed midwife she was not to deliver at home past forty-two weeks, so she started coming up with ways to encourage me to go into labor. My days became all about getting that baby out. I tried homeopathic remedies, herbal tinctures, chiropractic adjustments, walking uphill, getting my membranes stripped, taking castor oil, having sex. Nothing.

I was also going to the hospital every couple of days to check on the baby, which meant submitting to ultrasound, external fetal monitoring, and pressure to induce labor. The first of these ultrasounds was reassuring (fluid level fine, baby responsive, everything normal) and even exciting (surprise! despite the results of my first ultrasound, it's a boy in there after all. Michael's comment: I've never been so happy to see another guy's penis).

For a few days the whole baby-having thing was fun and exciting again. Then the days wore on, the anxiety returned, and the physician at the nonstress test station strongly recommended that I be admitted to labor and delivery for immediate induction. I had to face the possibility of a hospital delivery.

Many women have hospital births, I told myself, so why was I so worried? Well, first of all, I was used to having my babies at home and their births had been awesome experiences. I wanted to share that awe with my daughters, to give them the unique experience of witnessing the gentle and natural birth of their sibling. Suddenly, though, I was facing this other scenario and I had no time to prepare for it. I feared the intervention domino effect likely to follow hospital admission for induction: labor-inducing drugs, unnaturally hard contractions, supine position, fetal monitoring, epidural, episiotomy, or, quite likely, a failure-to-progress caesarean section. I dreaded the idea of fighting hospital protocol every step of the way as I am not always assertive enough. And deep down I still trusted my body. Part of me just wanted to go off and find a cave somewhere and do this on my own.

On Thursday, November twentieth, the midwives gave me a deadline of Saturday. I had tried many physical things; it was time to explore the metaphysical realm. I was on the phone with Shelly, and she asked what I thought might be holding me back. The only thing I could think of was Sarah. Sarah would be here on the twenty-fifth, and I had to admit that in the back of my mind I'd again begun to cultivate the hope that she would be at the birth. Shelly, however, made it clear that the baby needed to come before that, one way or another, so I would have to let go of that hope. (I've had to do a lot of letting go regarding Sarah's life.)

I called Sarah but got the machine, so I started having a conversation with her in my mind while I again prepared the bedroom for the birth. I laid out a baby outfit and put the plastic sheet back on the bed between layers of fitted sheets. Then I went outside and read with Zoe in the courtyard of our apartment.

After I while I felt a bit of a trickle between my legs. "I think my water just broke," I said to Zoe and went to spread the news to Michael, my mother-in-law, and my midwives, who gave me a new deadline of twenty-four hours. Zoe was so excited. So was I. When I was pregnant with Zoe, my water broke and within three hours there she was. Certainly this baby would be here before tomorrow.

Clear fluid soaked pad after pad throughout the night. But no contractions came, aside from the Braxton Hicks I'd been having throughout the pregnancy. The next thing I knew, it was morning and I was still pregnant.

I called the midwives, desperate. Even I was beginning to worry and doubt my body. Shelly told me that I had till noon or she'd take me to the hospital, and she asked me to ask my baby what it wanted. I felt frustrated and on the spot. I couldn't answer her, couldn't concentrate. I needed to be alone. I got off the phone and went for a walk.

When I was pregnant with Sarah, I was in an unhappy marriage, and I developed a special, desperate sort of connection to the baby inside me. When I was pregnant with Zoe, I was deep in grief over having Sarah taken from me, and I developed a special, desperate sort of connection to her. Now with this pregnancy I have a happy life. I realized that whenever I spoke or thought about having this child, it was always in terms of him joining our family. I would say: we want you to be born. I talked about a sibling for Zoe or a son for Michael.

As I walked uphill yet again, trying to bring on contractions, I had a tearful talk with my baby. I let him know that I wanted him, that I loved him, and that I was looking forward to mothering him. Then I told him to come out. Come on out now, I said, so I can see you and nurse you and hold you in my arms.

I came home and Shelly came over. She had me lie down, and whenever I felt a Braxton Hicks contraction, she inserted the long needle used for rupturing membranes. Though I had been leaking water, a fluid-filled bubble in the sac still blocked the way of the baby's head. While the midwife tried to maneuver her straight stick through the curved passageway, she encouraged my husband to stimulate my nipples. When she said he needed to be more aggressive about it, Michael asked Zoe to leave the room and he began sucking on them, hard. Still, nothing seemed to be happening, and I think the three of us were pretty nervous as we continued to work on my body like this for quite a long time. Michael, always one to use his wit to dispel tension, said that this wasn't exactly the way he had imagined having a threesome.

Finally, after much sucking, poking, and prodding, I started to feel real contractions. Hooray! Shelly phoned her assistant and apprentice while I walked around the courtyard with Michael. Leaning on him and moaning, I forced myself to keep walking, even during contractions. When they got stronger and more frequent (and I got louder), we came inside and walked around the dining room table.

It's weird being in labor in an apartment building in the daytime. I saw the manager in the courtyard and asked her to tell the repairman, who was on his way over, to come another day. A little later a package was delivered between contractions, and I had to share a laugh with my family after sending the guy on his innocent, oblivious way.

Soon I could no longer walk during contractions. I dropped down on all fours in the hall and told my other midwife, Seannie, that I needed to pee. She whispered to Shelly that I was probably ready to push. I got on the bed, and an internal check revealed that I was just a slight cervical lip short of full dilation. Seannie helped me with that on the next contraction, applying oil and wet compresses made from five-by-five-inch pieces of cloth kept warm in a Crock-Pot.

Zoe said that the baby was coming out and went to fetch her grandma. I told her I didn't I think it was quite time yet. I didn't want to get my hopes up. But she went anyway, and of course she was right: the head was right there crowning.

I struggled and searched for a good position. With my other babies I had been on my hands and knees, but this time I ended up more upright, with my knees on the bed and my arms around Michael, yelling in his ear. I felt the head come out then waited for the contraction that would bring the shoulders. When it came, I pushed and yelled, and I felt the shoulders slowly emerging. Instead of the rest of the baby just slithering right out, I had to keep pushing as the chest slowly worked its way through as well. The midwives encouraged me to reach down and get my baby. I touched him and out he came: beautiful, perfect, gorgeous, a nine-pound, ten-ounce boy, squeegeed clean by his tight-squeeze birth.

I didn't tear at all, and I couldn't believe how easy my recovery was. The midwives were absolutely amazing, taking such good care of me after the birth as well as before and during. I'm very glad I didn't have to go to the hospital, and I'm glad I didn't have to go find that cave, either. I'm grateful for this home birth, for Michael's help, for the presence of Zoe and her grandma, and for the kind, loving hearts and very skilled hands of my midwives.

We named our baby Holden Michael. He was born at 12:44 PM on Friday, November twenty-first. Sarah met him four days later.

Who knows why Holden was born later than we expected? Maybe he would have come when he was ready without all of our efforts and still have been fine, though I don't think I would have wanted him to get much bigger. Perhaps I was wrong about my dates or his was just a variation of normal gestation, forty weeks being an average. Maybe there was indeed something in my mental state holding him back. Maybe he wanted to be a Sagittarius instead of a Scorpio. Who knows?

I'm just happy everything turned out the way it did. And happy to be able to write this while holding my sweet precious son, Holden, in my arms at last.

~

RYAN AND BRIANNA DIRKS'S BIRTH STORY

RYAN: My beautiful wife, after eighteen hours becoming more and more the most amazing and powerful human being that I have ever known, finally lifts our little boy out of the water and onto her chest. Larger than life really, he looks huge, magnificent in our minds, which have been intensely focused on him for the last nine months, and now, God willing, for the rest of our lives.

BRIANNA: For me labor started three weeks beforehand. Every weekend it was: is this it? I would get so excited, only to have it be another false alarm. It had gotten to the point that I thought I would have to see our baby Tucker's face before I would believe that it was really labor.

RYAN: Three Fridays in a row we had hoped ourselves right into labor. The first time, about a week before his due date, the most powerful contractions that she had ever experienced wrenched her out of bed, but she went back to sleep, and I went to school, to wait anxiously.

I might as well been one of the thousands of relatives that had been calling for the past three weeks as I woke her up with the phone call, "Just, uh, making sure everything's okay." Finally my boss forced me out of the shop before I drove him up the walls with my edgy nerves.

I thought I had gotten it all out of my system. Now I could just relax, knowing that fretful anticipation would get us closer to mental breakdown, not to Tucker's birth.

But the next Friday I didn't even make it to school. This time the contractions were regularly five to ten minutes apart. This had to be it. After three hours of wondering whether or not this was it, we got out of bed and did a two AM house cleaning between contractions. After wearing ourselves out cleaning, we slept some more, we showered, we ate, we drank, and the contractions were still fairly regular, so we called our midwife, Veronica, just in time to miss all of my classes for the day.

"[It's] your body trying to get him moved around," she said. Not labor.

Another week passed, and we watched his due date come and go. We went to the final Bradley class without the baby to show off like we'd hoped.

And we moped. A week and a half later, Brianna went to get an ultrasound with Veronica to check that the placenta was holding up. All was well. Tucker was positioned perfectly, but if he waited much longer, the natural, home birth that we had hoped for would not be for Tucker, as Veronica would only deliver at home up to forty-two weeks.

BRIANNA: My due date came and went. At a week and a half overdue, we had to do a biophysical profile to make sure everything was still okay. I was starting to get nervous that we might end up having to deliver in the hospital after all. After all we had been through to have a home birth, it seemed so unfair to then have to go to the hospital after all.

RYAN: Didn't he know he was late for his own birthday? Lord knows we had tried to tell him. Brianna made birthday cookies, and he didn't show up for them. Brianna made birthday cupcakes, and he didn't show up for them. It became more and more difficult to keep frustration out of our conversations with the little ingrate.

After the "Tucker's a week and a half late and we're getting frustrated" ultrasound, we went to Veronica's for a meeting to discuss our options. We could look forward to another ultrasound every few days until someone finally insisted on an induction. Fighting with doctors was something that we'd hoped to be done with after firing the last one.

So what could we do? We tried sex, but apparently my stuff wasn't doing the trick quite as well as it had forty-one and a half weeks ago. We could strip the membrane and see if that release of prostaglandins would jump-start labor. Sure, let's try that. But, no, Tucker wasn't quite far enough down for Veronica to reach yet.

BRIANNA: After the ultrasound, we decided to take matters into our own hands and try castor oil. I was pretty nervous because of all of the horror stories that I had heard.

RYAN: What else? Castor oil. Hmmm. We'd heard about that stuff, mostly that it's disgusting. But Veronica said, "I've heard of people mixing it with ice cream and saying that it doesn't taste too bad." "And it'll work to get his little butt out here?" "It might." But it was sure better than sitting around, planning the next ultrasound.

So we left the appointment at Veronica's house excited at the "green light" to try castor oil. All things need to be planned, though, and we had to consider that Brianna needed some nutrition in her system before she went into labor. But castor oil sometimes has the side effect of emptying the stomach from the top, so it was best to eat and digest before taking the oil. But by the time we got home and fixed dinner, and in order for her to be far enough into labor to justify my missing the next day's test.... At any rate, we decided that a couple of hours after eating was enough time for digestion before she tried the castor oil. So we enjoyed a meal at a local Mexican restaurant. On the way out, we discovered—actually, she discovered with a quick trip to the bathroom—that she was having one of the infamous symptoms of starting labor: loose bowels. We had been fooled by those before, though, so next stop: Laxative Land.

Tidyman's did not turn out to be the place, but the conversation with the pharmacist, who herself was pregnant and therefore sympathetic to our plight, was sort of worth the stop. The grocery store, then, became the Promised Land, and after scoring the dope, we used some more of our digestion time with a trip to the video store.

There we chose one for fun: *Monsters Inc.*; one for "Ryan, you have to see this movie": *Save the Last Dance*; and one that I had heard was an artistic film worth seeing: *The Cook, the Thief, His Wife and Her Lover.* (It was definitely an artistic film, and it was definitely not worth seeing, in case you're curious.)

At home I fed the outside animals, and Brianna talked on the phone for a while, too long in my opinion. "Honey, let's focus here: we're trying to have a baby and soon, because that test is getting way too close for comfort."

So I started to prepare the shake. We had decided that more ice cream would be stretching our budget further than our dinner and the movies already had. (Obviously, we had not yet lost our ability to think logically.) The shake, then, would come from what we had in the freezer, cookies and cream ice cream. A CCC special: cookies and cream and castor oil, MMMM-mmmmm.

BRIANNA: We mixed the castor oil with a cookies and cream milkshake. What a mistake that was. I will never again drink a "cookies and cream" milkshake ...EEEEEWW!

RYAN: Too bad we ran out of ice cream, or I just couldn't have resisted using the rest of the castor oil to make myself one. Then I broke the blender. Actually, the blade was rusted into position, so the motor started burning up, and to make a longer story shorter, the shake was hand blended. And she downed it.

BRIANNA: I think I would have been better off just gagging down the castor oil. At least then I wouldn't have such a bad association with milkshakes. So that was at nine o'clock, and we decided to watch a movie, *Monsters Inc.*

RYAN: Apparently I was wrong in my assessment of how appealing the CCC shake would be. The grimace stayed on her face through half of *Monsters Inc.*, but she kept it all down, and I was utterly impressed, as I would be many more times in the next twenty-four hours.

After the movie, I had all but resigned myself to suffering through my test the next day. Neither of us had dared hope that this would work to bring the little one out, so we went to bed without talking about the chances.

BRIANNA: At eleven o'clock we tried to go to bed, but I started having pretty strong contractions.

RYAN: Brianna didn't stay in bed long and was up by eleven with stronger contractions than she had ever felt. They were about five minutes apart. "Aren't we supposed to start with, like, a half hour between them?" Apparently not, as they were definitely strong, stop-her-in-her-tracks contractions and consistently five minutes apart.

BRIANNA: I seemed to have skipped early first stage labor and went straight to the serious stage.

RYAN: We refrained from calling Veronica, however, fearing that she would again take away Tucker's birthday.

BRIANNA: I was still walking around and getting things ready with Ryan. We took a shower, we ate, we drank, and we cleaned …

RYAN: … but would have to stop and focus on relaxing during the contractions, stopping every five minutes to breathe deeply and focus, as we had learned to do from Dolores, our wise and wonderful Bradley instructor.

Cleaning was the big job. The kitchen was a mess, the birthing room still needed to be organized a bit, the pets needed to be moved to less distracting areas of the house, and all in five-minute spurts between forty-five-second intervals of her gut wrenching pain, which I did my best to be helpful through.

BRIANNA: Ryan would stop what he was doing and help talk me through each of them . . .

RYAN: . . . like a fly trying to give an eagle help to stay aloft.

At one o'clock in the morning we decided that there was no going back, no way Veronica could tell us that this wasn't it, but I still held my breath all the way through Brianna's phone conversation with her.

BRIANNA: I called Veronica, our midwife, at about one, and we talked on the phone through four or five contractions. At this point my contractions were about five minutes apart and lasting for about one minute. Veronica confirmed that I was really, truly in labor, so Ryan started filling up the birthing tub.

Veronica arrived at about three in the morning. During that time I called my mom, and she and my cousin Hilde started on their way down. I also called my dad, but he decided to wait until the midwife had arrived and checked me to see when he would come down.

It wasn't too long until the hot water heater ran out, so Ryan started boiling water on the stove to continue filling the tub. When he unhooked the hose from the kitchen faucet, he left the end of it in the sink. It fell out and drained all over the kitchen floor. (And we thought he was housebroken!) Also during this time, Ryan moved the birds to the extra bedroom, got Mister Kitty situated in the cat room, and did the last bit of cleaning that needed to be done.

Throughout this time I could still talk and move about between contractions, so I showed Veronica our wedding album.

At about five thirty AM, I lay on my side while waiting for the tub to be filled. I got in the tub fifteen minutes later. Heaven! It felt nice to be in the warm tub. It was easier to relax there, and I just felt more comfortable. Not too long after that, my contractions seemed to get stronger and I began moaning through them. When I got out of the tub to use the bathroom, the contractions felt

unbearable. I decided right then that I would rather be in the tub than anywhere else.

RYAN: I'd like to say that I did a wonderful job and all, but, really, the tub was
wonderful. True, I was there and helped her through the times that she had to
be out of the tub, but the difference was like night and day: when she was out
of the tub, I would be there for her saying, "Yes, we can do this; you're doing
great." In the tub she was in control and all about getting down to business,
focusing on what her body needed to do.

But if anything was a surprise about the labor, it was the moaning. It worried
me at first. "Whoa. Wait, that doesn't look like relaxing to me." And at that time
it wasn't, because she was resisting the urge to let it out. Veronica encouraged
her, though, by joining in the next time, matching her pitch, kind of singing
with her. After realizing that it was okay, it did become a relaxing technique.
When a contraction came on, it was like there was something building inside
of her, from deep within her soul, the nature, the strength of a woman. And it
showed itself during the contractions as the majestic crescendo of her voice.

BRIANNA: Dad and Lane arrived during this time. I was drinking Gatorade and
occasionally having some peaches that Mom and I had canned a few weeks earlier. Right around seven in the morning, I vomited up all of the peaches and
Gatorade. After that it was hard for anyone to get me to eat anything. I continued to drink, but now I just wanted tea.

At around ten thirty, they made me get up and walk around outside to try
to help move labor along. I remember that the cool air outside felt good after
sitting in the steamy birthing room for so long. But I had figured out my coping technique in the tub, and outside was different. When the contraction
came, I was standing up. I panicked and didn't know what to do. The contraction was so strong that I started breathing hard and crying.

Luckily, Ryan was there, and so were my mom and Hilde. They all held on
to me and helped me through the contraction. I leaned on Ryan with my arms
around his neck while Hilde and mom held me too.

Throughout this whole time Ryan never left my side, except to go to the
bathroom. Through every contraction he put counter pressure on my lower
back to help ease the pain. He moaned through the contractions with me. I
found that if I tried to get my moan lower like his, it helped more. The lower

and deeper my moan, the better I felt. In between contractions he told me how wonderful I was and how proud he was of me. There is no way I could have done it without him. His support and encouragement are what kept me going, even when I didn't think there was any way I would make it.

All I wanted to do was get back in the tub after that, but Veronica wanted to check me first, so we went to the bedroom. I was almost completely dilated except for a small lip of cervix, so Veronica asked if I wanted her to try to reduce it during my next contraction. I knew it might hurt, but I was more afraid that it might cause my labor to intensify. I didn't think I could handle contractions that were any stronger. Of course I wanted to be closer to done, but I was afraid. I eventually decided to go ahead and try. It was extremely difficult to relax while Veronica was doing it, and I felt scared, but it was over pretty quickly. I was grateful to go back to the tub after that.

So now I was complete. I could start pushing any time now. It was about noon. I was scared to push, so I decided to rest through some contractions and try a little bit later. I was so tired. I remember falling asleep in between contractions. I couldn't help it; I was so tired. I could tell that everyone was getting a little worried about me.

I still didn't want to eat anything, even though I knew that I probably should. They finally talked me into having a little bit of noodle soup. Ryan put a pillow on his lap so I could lay my head back between contractions.

Every once in a while, without my doing anything, my body would spontaneously push. It was scary and painful, like my body was a battering ram. It felt like my insides were slamming downward. If that was what it felt like to push, I wanted nothing to do with it. I felt so out of control when it happened. I tried pushing a little bit, but it hurt, so I didn't want to continue.

They wanted me to try different positions, so I tried being on my hands and knees for a few contractions. When I fell asleep between contractions, my face fell into the water. Besides, I didn't like that position; I just wasn't as comfortable. So they made me go outside again.

I was scared even before I was outside. I started to panic again as the contraction started, but with Ryan and my mom and Hilde's help, I got through it. I felt so vulnerable outside. I was thankful to get back to the tub.

At about three, Veronica sat down with me, and we talked about where I was and what was going on. I was getting very, very tired, yet I didn't want to push. In fact, I was scared to death to push. I was so afraid of losing control, I couldn't even think about pushing. I didn't want to scream; I didn't want to lose my cool. I was so afraid that if I let go of my composure, I wouldn't make it through.

With some encouragement from Veronica, I realized that no one was going to judge me if I lost control. I was safe. And even if I couldn't do it, no one would think less of me. Ryan wouldn't be mad; he would love me just the same. I decided that I wanted just Ryan and Veronica in the room while I was pushing. I needed at least that much control.

I decided that if I was going to push, I had better get as much done with each push as possible. Once I started, I realized that after the first push of each contraction (which hurt badly), the other pushes felt better.

It seemed like I had been pushing forever, so Veronica asked me if I could feel Tucker's head. I think maybe I did, but at the time I didn't realize it. When she had me check again later, I knew I felt his head, and I could feel it move down as I pushed. I became pretty excited, because I could finally tell that I was getting somewhere. It still seemed a lot slower than I had expected, but at least it was progress.

For the first part of pushing I just sat in the tub, but as I became more serious and pushed harder, I wanted my knees up and I wanted to be off my butt. I started to squat with my arms hooked through Ryan's. When I started pushing, I would pick my feet off the bottom of the tub and hold my knees up with my hands. Ryan was standing behind me, supporting all of my weight as I pushed. The whole time he kept encouraging me, telling me how well I was doing and how strong he thought I was and how proud he was of me.

After two hours of pushing, I finally felt Tucker's head crown. I remember thinking, "Ow, that hurts . . . finally!" It was an entirely different type of pain, sharper than the contractions and definitely more focused. But it was much easier to handle because I knew I was almost there. The hardest part was all that was left, and suddenly I knew I could do it. I kept my breathing shallow during these contractions so I wouldn't push too hard. I only pushed little teeny pushes as Veronica told me to so I wouldn't tear as badly.

I reached down to feel Tucker's head coming out, and it felt like a bowling ball was down there. I wasn't sure how he was going to come out, but I kept trying. Finally his head was born. I remember looking down and seeing lots of hair swaying in the water, just like I wanted.

I thought that it would be easy after that: he would just come sliding out. I was wrong. I still had to get his shoulders out. I was exhausted by this point and didn't think I could push any more, but with a few more good, strong pushes, he came out.

Veronica said to me, "Catch your baby." So I reached down and pulled him out of the water. He seemed so big. So huge and magnificent. And so purple! All I could say was, "Oh, my God! Oh, my God!"

I held him to my chest, and Veronica covered him with a receiving blanket. She suctioned his nose and mouth. About this time my whole family came piling through the doorway. Everyone was crying and saying how beautiful he was. Ryan cut the umbilical cord. Then Veronica told me to hand Tucker to Ryan so I could get out of the tub. I heard Ryan try to sing his song to the baby, but he couldn't because he was crying.

RYAN: No I wasn't... All right, maybe a little.

At any rate, I followed Brianna into the bedroom with our new baby boy. We collapsed on the bed, all three of us, exhausted from the last seventeen and a half hours of labor, and slept, waking gloriously rested in the morning to start our new life.

Sort of.

BRIANNA: Actually, after getting out of the tub, there was another two hours of work to do. First of all, I still had to deliver the placenta, and I had thought we were done pushing! That took a while, but at least it didn't hurt. Next we tried to nurse. I was a little nervous that we might have a hard time, but Tucker was a pro. He nursed for a half an hour straight. What a champ!

RYAN: Thus began our life as parents. It was beautiful to see my wife, after such an ordeal, calmly put her breast to our son's mouth and nurse him for the first time. It did take a few tries for him to "latch on" and begin eating, but Brianna was patient, Tucker was diligent, and everything came together after a short time.

The next half hour or so was a blur of excitement as Grandma Sue-Sue oiled Tucker's butt and diapered him in preparation for our introduction to meconium; the midwives administered some of the recommended precautions, then weighed and measured him; and we got down to the business of mending Brianna.

BRIANNA: Next we discussed my tears. I didn't want to hear about it, but oh, well. My mom and Hilde took Tucker out to the living room while I was being stitched. Three tears total. Two weren't so bad: a little bit of lidocaine and I was good to go. The third tear was a whole different story.

RYAN: The stitching was interminable. Without the job of pushing on Brianna's back, holding her up while she pushed, or getting to know our new baby (he had been taken from the room for the stitching procedure by Brianna's mom and cousin), the adrenaline was starting to wear off and I was about ready to pass out.

The third tear was questionable: it might heal on its own; it might require stitches. So we decided to consult a doctor the next day.

BRIANNA: So I had my glass of orange juice and some chicken and dumplings that, had I not been so hungry, I wouldn't have touched with a ten-foot pole. Funny what not eating will do for you.

Everyone was about to leave when I realized that I was kind of a mess. A shower was high on my list of priorities, so everyone hung out a bit longer. Sadly though, my shower with Ryan (for safety) was cut short when everything started spinning on me. I barely made it back to the bed before I blacked out momentarily. So a shower was not in the cards for me right then.

Oh well, there was always tomorrow.

RYAN: Finally, Veronica tucked all three of us tired souls into bed for the night. Oh blessed sleep! But that was not for long, either.

BRIANNA: We woke gloriously—actually sleepily—two hours later, as would be the trend for at least the first six months of Tucker's life, to start our new life as parents.

꿍

KARIN KEOGH'S BIRTH STORY

I HAD AN incident-free pregnancy, except for one day at about five months when I had a bit of spotting, which was very scary. Other than that all was well. I am a small-framed person (five foot, three inches and rarely over ninety-five pounds), so I started showing quite early, about four months if not before. I also became quite uncomfortable fairly early. Yoga was a savior in that respect; I would not have survived pregnancy without it.

I also felt Braxton Hicks contractions around four months and started leaking colostrum about that time. I remember the first time that I realized these were Braxton Hicks. I had been feeling the tightening for a while but had always assumed that it was the baby stretching or something. My sister Katie, who has two children and is a doula, liked to practice palpating my abdomen, and almost every time she did, especially around the top of the fundus, it would stimulate Braxton Hicks contractions. Throughout my pregnancy, I could not wear elastic waist bands above or on my stomach because they always stimulated contractions.

I was lucky enough to live near a freestanding birth center, an hour and fifteen minutes away. In my opinion, every woman should have the opportunity to give birth in a birth center. I cannot begin to say how important this is to me. I knew from the very beginning that I did not want a hospital birth—too many horror stories, too many interventions, too much to fight. I wanted and needed to be able to give birth in a warm, calm, supportive environment, and it helped to know that if a problem did arise, I was literally across the street from a good hospital.

I had decided long ago that I would have a drug-free labor, as natural as I could safely have. One huge reason the birth center was so appealing was that they will not give you pitocin or any analgesics during the birth. If you change your mind, you must be transferred to the hospital. This was not a concern to me. I knew I could do it naturally. My mother had four natural births, and my sister had two. Of course I could!

My favorite book during the pregnancy was *Gentle Birth Choices*. Every page made me feel so calm yet excited, very empowered, never apprehensive, about the upcoming birth. I read all I could get my hands on about birth centers and water birth. Oh, did I want a water birth! It made so much sense to me.

I planned to have my family present for the birth, basically whoever wouldn't be bothered by blood. I also reserved the right to kick everyone out if I changed my mind at the last minute, which, of course, they understood. Actually, when I spoke to my brother a few weeks before the birth, he sheepishly asked, "I don't *have* to watch the baby come out, do I?" "Of course not," I said. I found that pretty amusing.

So the chain of events was this:

On Thursday, October seventeenth, I had a prenatal appointment. The previous day I had started losing my mucus plug, and I was telling everyone. I told a complete stranger in the waiting room of the birth center, and she was excited for me; she told me about when she lost her mucus plug, down to times and everything. I knew that it could happen two weeks ahead of time, but I was excited anyway.

Saturday morning I woke up feeling strange. I went to my sister's room, crawled onto her bed with her, and said, "I'm hot, but I'm cold, I feel weird, and I want Mom!" and cried. I felt so young and weak all of the sudden. Our mother was planning to come up in the next couple of days to stay with us until the baby was born. Then my father and brother would come when I was definitely in labor. At the time, Mom was with our oldest sister Kristy, who had just had dental surgery. We called Mom at Kristy's and asked if everything was all right enough at Kristy's for Mom to come up now because I needed her, didn't have an explanation, just needed her. So she came. She arrived Saturday evening; I was so relieved just having her near. I felt 150 percent better. We had a relaxed evening: we just ate dinner and enjoyed each other's company.

On Sunday morning, there was a Renaissance festival. We had been planning to go with my brother-in-law Dean's family, and I thought, well, walking couldn't hurt. Not so secretly, I was ready to get this baby out. That morning I noticed a bit more mucus plug and little bit of blood. We decided to take an extra vehicle, so Mom could bring me home if I needed to leave early. We walked around for a while; I waddled slowly and had a good time. I was definitely in outer space though. After a couple of hours, we made our way to the stands where they were about to have a jousting tournament. We climbed almost to the top of the stands, and right about the time the stands were filled and everything started, I needed to get out of there. I felt too closed in. So

Mom and Dean helped me get out of the stands (that was a task!), and we made the long, long way back to the car. I remember just feeling weird. I wasn't having any cramps or contractions other than the Braxton Hicks I had throughout the pregnancy. I just felt so heavy. I was relieved to get back to the house. I think all we did the rest of the day was take a trip to the health food store to pick up a couple of last-minute food items for the labor just in case.

Monday about two in the morning, I woke with a deep soreness in my abdomen. It's strange; I didn't think "labor" at the time. I just kept moving around trying to get comfortable. I ended up on my knees, bent over with my head on the pillow; that felt pretty good. Then I realized that the soreness seemed to be coming and going, and it kind of felt like I was getting my period. Then it dawned on me: this must be it! I knew I should try to go back to sleep, but I couldn't; I was just too uncomfortable. I started walking around the house, seeing if that felt better, and I noticed it was better if I made a bit of noise during the contraction. The contractions were nothing like I was expecting. I didn't feel a tightening like with the Braxton Hicks, just a deep, low soreness coming then going. So I walked around, and whenever a contraction started, I would kind of bend and lean on something (like the kitchen counter) and moan through it. I was a bit hungry, so I made some toast and nibbled it between contractions.

By this time it was a little after three o'clock, I think, maybe four. I suddenly felt like I didn't want to do this alone anymore, so I woke my mother. Right after I woke her, I had another contraction and had to lean on the dresser for a moment, making noise because it helped, and she came over to me and rubbed my back. I was so happy to have her there. We wandered out into the house, and I shuffled around, having the occasional contraction. I think they were about five minutes apart this whole time but not necessarily regular. I think I was a little bit freaked out at that point. I knew it was very early labor, and I definitely needed to moan and work to get through each contraction. So my mind kept wandering to: how am I going to handle active labor? I finally had to just make myself stay in the moment, not think ahead to the next contraction, just think about them one at a time. It actually worked!

I think that set the tone for the rest of the labor because after that point I lost all concept of time. Not long after that, Katie and Dean joined us in the living room; I imagine my moans finally woke them. I think it was about five o'clock in the morning at this point. We talked and joked; it was still pretty relaxed.

Mom and Dean were taking turns writing down the times of my contractions, still about five minutes apart but not regular. I was starting to feel like things were progressing, though.

I think Katie was going around the house collecting things for the birth center, making sure we had everything ready, and preparing the car. Everyone was just letting me do my own thing. I decided that I wanted to call the midwife to tell her what was going on and that I wanted to leave for the birth center soon. I think my mother called her and put me on after the facts were out. I told her how I was feeling and that I'd like to come, and she said that would be fine, but if I was two centimeters or less, she was supposed to send me home. She wanted me to be aware of this because the drive was over an hour long. We discussed it and decided that if it was too early, we would just get a hotel room near the birth center for a few hours. I really wanted to go because with every contraction I felt such extreme pressure on my cervix. I didn't want to stay home too long and have the baby on the highway. So we woke Katie and Dean's girls, and we went on our way.

Getting into the car was interesting. Luckily it was a decent-sized SUV with lots of space in the back. It was filled with blankets and pillows, so I could prop myself up however I liked, to try to get comfortable. My mother climbed in the back with me, and Katie drove. Dean followed with the girls in Mom's car. I was expecting the drive to go on forever, but it didn't. Well, it did, and it didn't. Like I said, I lost all concept of time. I do remember that with every contraction I would almost yell, "It feels like the baby's coming out!" I was sure I was fully dilated and I was going to have the baby right there. Later Dean told us he could tell when I was having a contraction because about every five minutes he had to step on the gas to keep up.

We finally arrived at the birth center just as it became light out. Imagine my disappointment when the midwife Nancy checked me and I was six centimeters—better than two, but I really thought the baby was coming out and I was going to whip right through this. Nancy knew that I was planning a water birth, and she said I could get in the tub whenever I wanted. I had read much about water birth and many testimonials about that described how as soon as these women climbed into the tub, it was like a natural epidural. It wasn't for me, although it was better, I'll admit.

I'm not sure how long I stayed in the water, but I think it slowed down my labor a bit. Katie started trying to talk me into getting out of the tub and walking around to speed things up. Finally and reluctantly I agreed to get out. They wrapped a towel around me, Katie hooked my arm over her shoulder, and we started walking up and down the hallway. Katie's oldest daughter took my other arm and let me squeeze her hand for support. She was awesome.

I was having hard contractions at this point. I had to stop in the hallway and hang on to someone to get through them. I decided that I wanted something else but didn't know what, so we walked back to the room. Right as we got back, I suddenly started throwing up. Luckily Nancy got the trash can under me in the nick of time. I had been drinking lots of watered-down grape juice to keep hydrated, so I had something in my stomach when it happened. Afterward Katie smiled at me and said in a sing-song voice, "Transition!" I had heard that a lot of women throw up as a sign of transition, but I was hoping to be an exception.

I allowed the midwife to check my cervix after that; I wanted to know how dilated I was. The vomiting episode had upped me to eight centimeters! My water had not yet broken, so she asked me if I wanted her to do that. I decided to let her, hoping that would speed things up a bit. This is when she told me that she saw a slight meconium staining in the water, which meant that legally I could not have a water birth. I was sort of disappointed, but I understood and didn't care. I think my mind was shutting down so my body could work. Things get blurry from this point.

I remember squatting at the side of the bed, with Katie behind me rubbing my lower back. I did that for a long time. I think I walked around here and there too. I remember going to the bathroom to pee and my body started pushing by itself. That was a weird feeling; I didn't know what was going on. I guess I was making a lot of noise because Nancy called into the bathroom saying, "You're not pushing, are you?" I remember that it was the only thing that felt good.

I can't remember when I was checked and told that I was completely dialated. I do remember asking if I could push now, and she said of course. I wanted to give birth squatting if I couldn't have a water birth. The idea of using gravity made a lot of sense to me. I knew that the only thing I didn't want was to give birth flat on my back. So I started pushing. I think this was around eleven in the morning. I just squatted at the side of the bed with Katie behind me for support. Pushing was the weirdest thing yet. I waited for a good, big contraction to begin, started pushing, and my body took over for the rest. It was bizarre. I understand how that feeling could be scary because you are not in control at that point. That was fine for me. I was in the zone. I did have to take over a bit toward the end of the contraction to keep it going. It was hard and tiring. It did feel good in a way though, like I was getting somewhere, like I wasn't fighting the contractions anymore; I was using them.

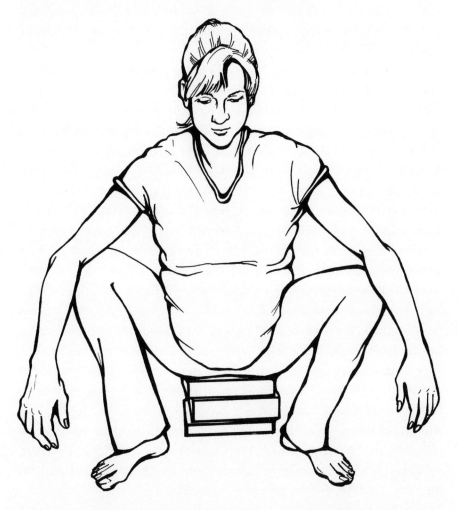

SQUATTING opens the female pelvis up to 30 percent. Instead of squatting freely, one can squat on a birthing stool or a pile of books. When used in pregnancy, labor, and birth, squatting helps a woman open her pelvis, allowing more space for the baby to maneuver and enabling her to see her baby come out. Forceps, vacuum, and caesareans need not be the preferred method for women with small hips to deliver larger babies. When the pelvis opens up with a simple squat and when the force of gravity, the uterine contractions, and the woman's pushing efforts are synchronized, it is possible for babies who would otherwise have been exposed to instrumental or surgical delivery to be born vaginally.

Things started to get a bit crappy at this point. I was pushing and pushing and nothing seemed to be happening. I was using all the visualization I could, and the baby just wouldn't slip right out like I had imagined so often. The other problem I was having (and, yes, this could have been all in my head) was that it seemed like after every push the midwife would sigh and look upset, like it was just not going to happen, this baby was never coming out. This really affected me. I did have times of encouragement: after a little while I could feel the top of the baby's head, and of course Katie and my mother were incredibly encouraging. I would have given up without them.

I kept changing positions, walking a bit more, hanging on people, things like that. I know that sometime around then I started giving my mother looks like: why can't you help me? I don't think I said anything; I just pleaded with her with my eyes. I think I occasionally said, "Mom, I'm so tired," and she would hold me up and say, "I know." I knew there was nothing she could do. I was completely on my own with this. Now I believe that that was something I had to mentally go through. I needed to realize that I had to—and could—do this.

I think it was about two and a half hours after I started pushing that Nancy suggested transferring to a hospital to get a Pitocin drip. The birth center midwives can allow you to push for only three hours before transferring. I gritted my teeth and said, "donwannahearit." Half an hour later she suggested it again, and I repeated, "donwannahearit." I was adamant about having my baby drug free in a birth center. At this point I was—surprise!—flat on my back in a bed, the only position I didn't want to use. I had no strength left to be in any other position. I had to use all my energy to push. I also had an intravenous drip to keep hydrated. Finally Nancy said that she would give me half an hour to keep pushing but then we would be transferring. Thirty minutes came and went, and I finally agreed. Mom made me feel better about it, telling me that she needed a pitocin drip with my brother because the same thing happened with him and she just needed that extra oomph to get him out.

I was lying there, four hours after the pushing started, still having contractions, pushing when they felt big enough and resting if they were smaller, while the midwife filled out the necessary paperwork for transferring. I was lying there thinking: how am I going to go from this bed, having contractions, across the street to the hospital, to a room, and so on and so on? I was thinking: let's just go and get this over with! That's when one of the other midwives, Kathy, came into the room.

She talked to me and Nancy and found out what was going on, and she said something like, "Did you try the 'something-something' stirrups?" We hadn't, so she pulled out these two separate strap things, a stirrup on one end and a handle on the other. They put them on my feet and gave me the handles, and when the next contraction came, I pushed with my body and pulled on the handles as hard as I could, and lo and behold, a head started coming … and coming … and coming, and I kept pushing, and everyone was yelling, "Come on! The baby's coming! Keep pushing!" and I kept taking more breaths and kept pushing, and I could feel the baby finally coming out. Then I heard someone yell, "It's a boy!"

There he was on my chest. I cried and cried and cried, and everyone around me was crying. He cried a little bit, and I shushed, trying to calm him, but they told me to just let him cry for a second. I found out later that he was a little purple when he came out, and they wanted him to suck lots of air into his lungs. He stopped crying by himself anyway. He had hardly any blood on him and no gunk of any sort. The next thing I noticed, other than how perfect and beautiful he was, was that he had an enormously large cone head. That's why it looked like he was coming and coming; it was all his head. Apparently it became misshapen from being in the birth canal for so long. I was assured that it would return to a normal shape very soon. I didn't care; he was perfect.

The time after his birth was also a blur, this time a wonderful blur. I found out that the person who called out "It's a boy" was my mother. It wasn't long before he tried suckling. We just lay there in the bed for hours. I'm not sure how long I held him before he was weighed and measured, but Finally it was announced that he was eight pounds, fourteen ounces and twenty-one and a half inches long.

Unfortunately it wasn't all wonderful after the birth, with me anyway. My uterus was so tired that I hemorrhaged a bit, and they had to give me Pitocin to get it to contract and stop bleeding. (The birth center couldn't give Pitocin during labor because that is an intervention, but could give it after the birth to stop the bleeding.) The midwife also had to firmly palpate my uterus to help it contract and to get any blood clots to come out; that was excruciating. I can honestly say that was the most painful part of the whole experience. But the bleeding stopped, and I delivered the placenta, which felt like nothing.

After several hours in bed, I finally stood up to try walking to the bathroom and was immediately woozy. When I caught a glimpse of myself in the mirror, it was terrifying! I didn't recognize myself. My face was swollen until almost perfectly round and it was white and gray and a little black and blue. I had gotten to the bathroom with help but almost passed out on the way out the door. I had lost a lot more blood than I realized. Instead of making me walk and pass out, people put a blanket on the floor, laid me down on it, and dragged me across the floor back to the bed. I thought it was a great idea!

A little while after that they made a bath for me in the huge tub, and I languished in it for a little while. I considered bringing the baby in with me but felt too weak, so I asked my mother to hold him in my line of vision so I could relax in the tub. I didn't want to take my eyes off him. It was wonderful. My sister washed my hair for me, and I felt fabulous.

The other occurrence was that my blood pressure rose after the birth, so I had to stay at the birth center longer than is usual so they could keep an eye on me, with a trip to the hospital threatened again if my blood pressure wasn't down by a certain point. Mom stayed with me so everyone else could go home and go to bed.

This was sometime way after dark. We tried to sleep, but I was too excited from the whole experience. I just wanted to lie there and talk. I snuggled the baby and practiced nursing. Finally my blood pressure lowered enough that it was deemed safe to send us home. In the days that followed, I was still having trouble with my blood pressure, and I was put on medication for a while. But the situation didn't last, and I was able to wean off of the blood pressure medication, and all is well.

And my son is still perfect.

⟨∽⟩

CHARLOTTE RUSSELL'S BIRTH STORY

IT TOOK ME eighteen months and two miscarriages to conceive my first son. Needless to say, I was a little wary of going down that road again. But I wanted another child.

In April, when Samuel was thirteen months old, we decided to start trying to conceive again. My husband didn't want to go through the same stress that I had experienced the last time, so we were supposed to be taking a laid-back approach this time around. Still, I knew when I was ovulating, and I was very good about initiating things during those three to five fertile days.

On August second, I suspected that I might be pregnant. In the middle of the afternoon, I took a test, which was negative. My period wasn't even due yet. Later I went back and looked at the test, and there were two lines. I decided to take another test. I took another, and it was positive within the given time frame. Before the weekend was over, I had four positive pregnancy tests. And before the week was out, I had lost yet another pregnancy.

We just couldn't go down this road again. We decided to let things be until the end of October. If I were not pregnant by then, we would opt for one of us to be sterilized and consider looking into adoption someday. I was planning to pursue a career in midwifery and started to work toward that end.

At the end of October, I was expecting a period. When I had ovulated, I was been late by a few days, so I wasn't surprised when my period didn't arrive right on time. That week I was painting the living room with a friend and mentioned that I felt tired and sick. I thought I had the flu. My friend begged me to take the last pregnancy test I had in the bathroom, telling me she'd buy me another if it were negative. So at two in the afternoon on November fifth, I took the test. It was positive.

I expected to be elated when I found out I was pregnant again, but I was filled with concern and trepidation. I had all of these plans laid out, and now they were going to be put on hold for a year. It took quite a while to get used to that idea, but once I heard baby's heart beat at ten weeks, I was sold on the idea of being a mom to two.

This time around I opted for a midwife, the one I had planned—and still do plan—to train with. Her birth center was one and a half hours away, and we dutifully drove there for every prenatal visit. It was a mercy that she felt I was healthy enough to come only every two weeks, at the end of my pregnancy.

I knew I was due sometime between July tenth and fifteenth, but hadn't anticipated being overdue. Samuel was born six days before his due date, and for some reason I expected about the same of Atley. Needless to say, by the time the fourteenth rolled around, I had realized that what they say about pregnancies is true: every pregnancy is different. Obviously, this baby wasn't going to be early.

At four thirty in the morning I woke, needing to pee, and realized that for the first time in weeks I had been sleeping soundly for more than four hours. I felt rested and thought to myself, "I'll never get back to sleep," as I crawled out of bed to head for the bathroom. It wasn't until I stood up that I realized I was also having a contraction, which wasn't unusual. As I walked into the bathroom, my water broke.

This was not how I wanted my labor to start. I wanted to labor with my water intact for so many reasons this time: the smell of amniotic fluid nauseated me after a while, the pain of having a baby's head against your cervix without the cushion of the water, the restrictions that result when your water breaks early (in the hope of preventing infection). Oh, well. There was nothing I could do about it now.

I decided to call Sylyna, my midwife, before I woke Jason up. After all, it could be a while before my contractions started or became regular, and he'd need his sleep. At four forty-five, Sylyna called me back, sounding groggy. I still hadn't had another contraction, so I had no idea what to tell her except: "My water broke, and it's clear." She asked me to wait thirty to forty-five minutes to assess the contractions before we decided what to do. Because Sylyna isn't licensed as a midwife in my state, the plan was to drive across the border to her home state and birth at her birth center.

After about three contractions, which were each around three to five minutes apart and lasting only thirty to forty-five seconds, I decided that I wanted to get on the road. I didn't want to wait forty-five minutes and end up riding an hour and a half with very intense contractions in our Ford Explorer with its very stiff suspension on Louisiana's horrible roads. I called Sylyna back and told her that I'd feel more comfortable if we could go ahead and get on the road. She agreed with me. By this time Jason was awake, so I asked him to call his grandparents to come and stay with Samuel until he woke up. I took a shower, ate a bagel (which took great determination because I kept forgetting about it), and grabbed a few last-minute things while we waited for Nana and Granddad to show up.

We got out of the house about five thirty in the morning, but still needed to stop for gas, some juice, and a snack. I had my first contraction in the car while Jason was inside the gas station paying for the gas, and I wanted to turn around and go home. It was going to be a long ride. After we got on the road, I told Jason that I wanted to time two or three contractions, then turn the car's clock off so we didn't go crazy. The contractions were three to five minutes apart, still lasting thirty to forty-five seconds each.

The drive was uneventful, except for the standard "you don't need to speed, honey" conversations. I didn't want to get pulled over because, first, it would have been inconvenient and, second, they were likely to want to escort us to the nearest hospital, someplace I did not want to be.

As we neared the birth center, I found myself thinking in terms of how many more contractions I had to deal with in the car. It helped a lot, since by now I was feeling a lot of pain in my back and I could feel the pressure of my cervix effacing. When we got there, I forced myself to let Jason take a picture, since I had no pictures of myself pregnant with this baby.

Tina, Sylyna's apprentice, met us at the birth center and told us that another mama's water had broken that morning as well. She was also planning a birth center birth, which really threw a wrench into my plans. I let her check me so we could come up with a course of action. I kept telling myself, "As long as I'm four to six, I'll be okay." I was four centimeters and eighty percent dilated.

At this point, the implications of the other woman's water breaking hit me. I wanted to leave and come back another day, in all honesty. The birth center is a two-story house with a living room, half bathroom, kitchen, and breakfast (now birth pool) room on the first floor and two bedrooms and a bathroom on the second floor. There's not a lot of space there, and I was worried about my privacy. I hadn't anticipated two women being in labor at once because it just doesn't happen. I found out later that she and I were the first people it happened to in four years.

I called a friend to express my concerns and must have looked quite the sight talking on the phone while standing outside the birth center in wet shorts (the baby was still high enough that water was leaking around him during contractions), and pausing so often to cling to the fence during a contraction. I was worried that I didn't have enough clothes because I hadn't expected anyone to be there besides the midwives and me. I didn't have any underwear not only because I don't wear underwear when I am pregnant, but also because I planned to wear the stretchy postpartum underwear home. I was kicking myself for being so careful not to pack too much and packing too little as a result. My friend was very understanding and concerned that I was going to let this slow down or stall my labor. She offered to drive the hour and a half to bring me some clothes to labor in and to act as doula for me if I needed it. I said I'd call her back after I talked to Jason.

I guess Jason was talking to Tina about my concerns while I was on the phone outside because when I was finished, she met me outside and asked if everything was okay. "No," I answered tearfully. I was disappointed, concerned, and worried that the other mama would get in the pool before I could do so, or that I'd keep the other mama from getting to use the pool during her labor. Tina assured me that we could maintain our privacy and that everything would be okay. At that point the other mama and her four teenage sons pulled up. I was not reassured.

Later Sylyna came to my room and said that the other mama was only dilated to two centimeters, so she had been sent out to have breakfast and told to take her sons home because they could not stay. I didn't see her for the rest of my stay at the birth center.

I retreated to my room, as my contractions were getting pretty strong and I didn't want to "lose it" in front of this family that I didn't even know. My friend whom I had asked to take pictures showed up, and she, Jason, and I sat in the room and chatted between contractions. By now the contractions were strong enough that they required my full attention and Jason's help to get through them. I tried lying down to rest a little but quickly found that I had to jump up every two minutes for a contraction. Standing up was just about the only position in which the pain in my back was tolerable.

At about nine thirty in the morning, we asked Tina to check me again. (I don't remember why.) I was still at four centimeters and eighty percent dilated. This was immensely disappointing news, since I felt like I'd been working so hard all this time. After she checked me, I tried yet again to urinate, I think partly to escape to the privacy of the bathroom. I knew that I needed to pee, but every time I sat on the toilet, another contraction would start. In the bathroom I had four contractions one right after the other, and the intensity changed so drastically that I screamed for Jason to get in there and help me.

He and Tina came running, and during the next few contractions I clung to Jason while Tina applied counterpressure to my back. I wasn't sure it was helping but wasn't sure it was hurting, so I didn't ask her to stop. Tina said that the change in intensity was probably because she had just checked me, and I resolved not to let her check me again until I simply couldn't cope with the contractions any more. I changed into my nightgown, since the belly panel on my now drenched shorts was getting very uncomfortable.

The bathroom wasn't air conditioned, and I was hot while I labored in there but felt trapped by the contractions, which were right on top of each other. When we managed to get back into my room, I stood in front of the air conditioning unit for every contraction. Poor Jason was freezing, but I was more comfortable there.

At about eleven in the morning, I couldn't stand the contractions any longer and asked again to be checked. I had tried resting, sitting, standing, using the birth ball—nothing was working. I wanted to be in the water, but the midwives wanted to see some change in my cervix before I got in the tub. I knew intellectually that I didn't want to get in the water at only four centimeters because it could stall my labor, but my intellectual was not in control at the time.

This time Sylyna checked me, and I was at five centimeters and eighty percent dilated. Again all that work and not much progress. I was starting to feel very defeated, and I think I mentioned that this was too much like Samuel's labor, in which I had labored while on Pitocin for twelve hours and had only dilated to three centimeters. Everyone assured me that this was not Samuel's labor and that I was making progress. Sylyna still didn't want to let me use the water because she didn't want things to slow down. I got kind of ugly at this point and said something to the effect of "That tub is the only reason I'm here, and if you won't let me use it, I should have stayed at home." I also promised to get out of the tub if my contractions slowed down. She relented and went to get the tub ready.

At eleven thirty, I got in the water and was surprised at how much help it wasn't. A friend of mine had told me that her contractions had become ten percent more bearable when she labored in water. This wasn't the case for me, although the next few contractions did come a little bit further apart, making me worry that I'd have to get out because they slowed down. I actually remember praying that they wouldn't slow down or spread out because I really liked the water, even if it wasn't the magic cure-all that I had anticipated. I think the answer to my prayer was a resounding, "Okay, Charlotte, you get your way."

It was harder for me to get on top of contractions when I was in the pool. What worked for one contraction wouldn't work for the next, and I found myself almost thrashing around during them, going from being on my back with a jet aimed straight at my sacrum, to being on my stomach (and no jets better be aimed at my belly!), to squatting in the middle of the pool, to sitting tailor style. One of those positions would usually work, but going through all of them to find that one position was causing my contractions to be more painful. After a while I was again at the point where I needed help to get through every contraction, and Jason didn't seem quite sure how to help me. I didn't know what I wanted, and I'm pretty sure I told him that more than once. I also remember saying that I should have taken my chances with the epidural. I knew better than that because the epidural didn't work with Samuel and only made things worse, and the midwives were kind enough to remind me of that.

Tina stepped in and told me that when I started to lose hold over the contraction, she wanted me to open my eyes and lock them with either Jason's or hers. I tried looking at Jason, but he seemed a little unnerved by it, so during the next contraction, I turned to her. She didn't let my eyes go and breathed with me through every contraction. After a few like this I again started to lose it. I was feeling a lot of pressure, but not pushing pressure. I remember that Atley was moving during contractions, something he did during the Braxton Hicks contractions all through my pregnancy, and I kept yelling, "Why's he moving?!" It made the contraction much more intense.

Sylyna noticed that I was starting to bear down at the peak of the contractions and asked if she could check me again. For about five minutes, we argued about this because I was scared to death that I'd still be a five or continue my earlier progression and be only a six. I finally conceded and agreed to let her check me, but then had two double peak-contractions only a few seconds apart. I went from crying, "What if I'm only a six?" to "They'll never stop long enough for you to check!" Finally she managed to check and found that I was completely dilated and ready to push if I wanted to. I always expected that to be a relief, but it was no such thing. I didn't want to push; I just wanted to have a baby.

At this point I contemplated asking the midwives to transport me to the hospital for a caesarean section—oh, the crazy things you think during labor—but decided that it would require me to endure too many contractions, not to mention the pain of the surgery afterward. I shored myself up for the task of pushing this child out.

It took a while to find a comfortable position for pushing, but I finally felt that a supported squat in the tub would let me push most effectively. My feet were against the wall of the pool and Jason supported my weight by holding my hands. I was concerned that it was too much for him because at one point I could feel his arms shaking. I think that for him, the hardest part was that I'd lean back and nearly fall asleep between contractions, leaving him to support my dead weight. I asked a few times if we needed to find a different position but then silently rejoiced when he said he was okay.

I didn't realize until I'd pushed for a while that the baby would be born into the water, and I think I remember asking if he was really going to be born in the pool. When the answer was yes, I told Jason that I was sorry he wasn't going to get to catch, but I wanted to bring baby up out of the water. He had really enjoyed catching Samuel and was looking forward to doing the same with this baby.

I also remember yelling at Jason as the baby started to crown that I never should have married someone who weighed more than nine pounds at birth.

Soon after, Atley's head was born. After his head turned, causing me to yell at him again for moving during a contraction, I said, "Okay, now for the shoulders." He was born with the next contraction, and I pulled him out of the water. As I held him to my chest, he reared back, lifted his head up, and looked around the room. At this everyone ooohed and aaahed over his size and strength, but he looked small to me.

Once again, I proved to be a very bad judge of the size of my child. I thought he was smaller than Samuel's nine pounds, four ounces, but he turned out to be nine pounds twelve ounces, a full eight ounces larger!

〰️

ANGELA MILLER'S BIRTH STORY

AND SO IT began that fateful evening. I went to the bathroom, and after I urinated, my body released some more liquid. I thought it felt strange, but it never occurred to me that my water was breaking. This was two weeks before the baby's due date, and I had gone upstairs to pack for our trip to the hospital. After much discussion and compromise, my husband Clint and I decided to have our baby with midwives in a birthing center adjacent to a local hospital. This felt like a good decision, given that I was interested in birthing at home and he was not. It couldn't have been a better choice for us.

I had imagined my water breaking as sort of a gush falling from me into a big puddle on the floor while I was grocery shopping or something. But this was different, so I decided to phone Ana, the midwife on call. I explained that I was releasing liquid in spurts and thought I should let her know. She said it was difficult for her to tell over the phone if my water had broken; the only way she could really be sure was to see me.

The hospital was thirty minutes away, and my husband was working a night shift, so I decided to stay at home and see if anything progressed. That was about eight o'clock in the evening. I called Clint, encouraged him to stay at work, and assured him that I would call if anything happened.

Shortly afterward, I started to feel light-headed and a little strange, so I went downstairs to watch a movie. As I was lying on the couch, I began having difficulty concentrating. Soon I was unable to stay focused on the screen. I remember thinking, "I feel too weird. This is it; this is definitely it."

I picked up the phone and began to call my mother, my father, my sister, and my midwife. During my conversation with Ana, the contractions started getting heavier. She stayed with me over the phone, and asked me to come in.

My memory is somewhat fuzzy, but I remember laboring at home alone for a while when suddenly Clint walked in the door. He saw the state I was in and began running around, getting things together. He then headed out to the store because I was determined to have these special LifeSavers to eat during labor. I realized that we were unprepared and hadn't packed a bag. We thought we had plenty of time before our due date. He was back in a flash with Recharge juice, tropical source wild cherry LifeSavers, and fruit.

We went upstairs, and I began writhing in pain. I remember very little about this time except rolling around on the floor and holding on to the bed, Clint lying beside me, a blank stare on his face. I think both of us were shocked that it was really happening.

From the time I found out I was pregnant, I had wanted a natural birth. I have never been more determined and more scared about anything in my life. Why scared? Sadly enough, there is so much negativity surrounding birth, especially in the United States. I had bought into those notions my whole life, almost to the point that I didn't know if I wanted to have children. I knew that giving birth was going to be the hardest thing I would ever do, especially if I did it naturally. I had done so much research and reading, eventually concluding that a natural birth was best for my baby and me.

During the nine months of pregnancy, I felt stressed because I didn't know if I had what it takes to give birth without drugs. I wanted to do that more than anything. I wanted my baby's first experience of the world to be the best it could be and so I wanted her to enter into it as purely and naturally as possible. This being so, I was also very nervous about going to the hospital too early for fear of intervention. So that night I wasn't sure when to leave the house. But at about midnight, the pain was intense. I said to Clint, "Let's go."

Only a few hours had passed, but it felt like forever. We rode to the hospital in total silence. I was gripping the seat, unable to speak. We arrived at one in the morning and pulled up to the front, forgetting that it was after hours and the door was locked. It was freezing cold, and I can remember falling down into the grass with a contraction. We made our way to the emergency entrance, but it was quiet. It was as if no one was around. We found our way to the elevator and rode up but to the wrong floor. It felt like we were in a maze. After finally reaching the birthing floor and after many contractions, I was brought in to a room and placed on a table. I was in so much pain that I didn't care what happened.

The nurse checked me and said I was dilated to four centimeters. I felt very discouraged. I thought, "After all this I still have six centimeters to go?" Ana arrived promptly, comforted me, and took me to my room. I felt so safe and cared for with her. She and the hospital nurses that night were the reason we had the birth experience we did. Clint asked her if she should get an epidural ready, just in case, and she said to him, "What?!? We're about to have a baby!"

She dimmed the lights and drew my bath. I stepped in and instantly felt relieved. The warm water soothed me entirely. I moved around in the bath for quite a while and remember holding Ana's hand. Ana herself had a home birth with her son, and I remember asking her how she had done it. She said to me, "Just like you are." In that moment I felt what so many women have felt before me: I am not alone, I am part of the whole, and I can do this. And I did.

She had left me to labor alone in the bath when I suddenly felt the uncontrollable urge to push. I remember grunting loudly as Ana peeked in, looking surprised, asking me if I was pushing. I looked at her and said, "I think so." She asked me to get out of the bath so she could check the dilation, then quickly announced, "We're ready to push!" It was three o'clock in the morning. I began to walk around that room like a wild woman, moaning and naked, throwing off my robe. I did not want to be touched, nor did I want any music or candles. I was on a mission and the mission was: get the baby out!

After kneeling, squatting, and being on all fours, I stood on the bed and pushed with all my might, with everything I had and everything I didn't have, with one hundred percent and then some. You hear stories about birth in which the baby just slides right out or about women who are in such good shape that they don't need to push. Well, not me. I pushed with more than I knew I had, and at seven minutes after four in the morning, our daughter Alyssa was born.

She came into the world without making a sound, eyes wide open and curious, looking around. We looked at her amazed, so in awe that we didn't even know if she was a boy or girl until finally one of the nurses asked us. Clint investigated and said, "It's a girl!" Words cannot describe the joy we felt. She was immediately placed on my chest and remained there for hours afterward.

Everything went well, and my family and friends stopped by to visit. I felt good and was ready to go home right away. We asked the doctor if we could have an early discharge and he agreed, saying that everything looked fine. We were home in our own bed by eight that night.

Looking back, there isn't a thing I would change. We had the birth experience that was just right for us. After all was said and done, I was even glad we chose the hospital for the birth because deep down I knew I would feel safer there. I am proud of myself, because even though all the interventions were available to me, I never asked for them. I suppose I was so committed to having a drug-free birth that somewhere inside of me I had the confidence and the faith to do it. As my husband likes to say, "She didn't even pop an aspirin." It was true; I was so filled with the warm and fuzzy feelings produced by my body's natural endorphins that I didn't need a thing.

Everything I needed was right there in front of me, nestled sweetly in my arms.

Courtney Crow Wyrtzen's birth story

Fiona's birth story began four months after the birth of her sister, Blythe. My pregnancy and birth with Blythe had been standard. It was a planned pregnancy during which I took prenatal vitamins; tried to eat the right foods; and attempted to exercise. I took a childbirthing class, spent early labor at home and went to the hospital after my water broke. I labored through the middle of the night for fourteen hours, first with my husband, then with several family members, in a big labor, delivery, and recovery room. I pushed for over an hour in the lithotomy position with little progress, and ended with a forceps-assisted delivery that ushered in a beautiful baby girl in the late afternoon of a Monday in March.

I was ecstatic to have a healthy baby and to have made it through the birth without incident. I had not had any pretense about even trying to have a natural birth. I had not taken a natural childbirth class. I had not researched alternative birthing ideas or methods. I had even pooh-poohed my friends who did these things and who hired doulas for their hospital births.

When Blythe was four months old, I read a book by Naomi Wolf titled *Misconceptions: Truth, Lies and the Unexpected on the Journey to Motherhood.* That book opened my eyes to a world I had never even considered: alternatives to the mainstream medical model of obstetrics and hospital birth. I was floored. How come no one had told me about this before? Then it hit me: I hadn't been ready. Indeed, many people had tried to expose me to ideas about natural childbirth on several occasions. Images flashed through my mind: my sister-in-law five years before, discussing her desire for a home birth with a midwife and a birthing tub; early in my pregnancy, one of my student employees handing me a book by Robbie-Davis Floyd called *Birth as an American Rite of Passage*, of which I read a few pages and said no thanks; friends discussing their Bradley classes and the risks of medication. But I was not ready to take in any of that; it was too far out of my experience.

Initially I was happy with my first birth experience. Then I began to see it more clearly: that my labor had stalled after I rushed to the hospital although I had been progressing just fine in the comfort of my home; how I had depended so much on the staff and not taken responsibility for educating myself or hiring a doula to assist us; how immobile I had been from the epidural; how hungry I was as I watched friends and family munch on food throughout my labor; how tired I became trying to push a baby out from a prone position; how very worn out and battle-weary I was when it was all over.

I will never forget the picture of my husband and me after the birth: me sitting on the bed wearily holding our new baby and my husband deflated on a lounge chair. The labor, delivery, and recovery room looked like a train wreck had blown through, with supplies all over the room, stirrups discarded to the side, crash cart along the wall, and forceps on the floor. There had to be a better way.

After I waded through the blame game ("Oh it must've been the doctor; *he* didn't educate me"; "It had to be the first nurse; *she* offered the epidural instead of helping me get into the shower"; "No, wait, it was my partner; *he* didn't know what he was doing"), I realized that the destiny of my first birth experience had been shaped largely by my own choices, and my ignorance had not helped. I knew that another path had been forged generations before me. It was my responsibility to find it for myself.

So Fiona's birth story began before she was even conceived, late one night in October. Later I realized that I was newly pregnant, but I was so newly pregnant that the pregnancy test did not even test positive. I threw the pregnancy test in the trash, knowing it was wrong. I felt pregnant. I could sense the presence of another taking shape in my body. I dug the test out of the trash twenty minutes later and saw the faint line that meant positive.

I called the obstetrician who had delivered Blythe eight months earlier to discuss treatment for a yeast infection. I was asked, "Are you pregnant?" I said, "No. I don't know. I don't think so. Well, you see I took a pregnancy test and it was negative . . ." "Yes?" "But when I went back to the trash later and dug the test out, it was positive." I was told: "You'd better come in." So I did. But in the back of my mind I knew two things: I was indeed pregnant and I was not interested in having the obstetrician's staff confirm the pregnancy because I was not going to have this baby through their office.

I walked out of the doctor's office with a positive pregnancy test in my hand and several questions in my head: Where would I have this baby? Where do I begin? Whose hands will he or she ease into just nine or so months from now? Do I have what it takes to even attempt natural childbirth? In the end, the answers to my questions took shape halfway around the world in the home of my sister-in-law, the one who had wanted a home birth with a midwife, maybe even in a birthing tub. She was now five months pregnant. In her home in Morocco, she had several key books that would begin the formation of my new birth experience. There I found a book about spirituality and its connection to pain-free childbirth and a fascinating if slightly patronizing book by a kindly older gentleman named Robert Bradley, who believed in replicating the birth environment of mammals for better birth outcomes. I devoured the books and discussed natural childbirth at length with my husband, Joel, his brother Jonathan, and his beautifully pregnant wife, Leslie.

I decided to search out a birthing center in my hometown. At that time, home birth was not an option because it would definitely have been way out of my comfort zone. I chose a popular birthing center about ten miles from my house.

After my first prenatal appointment at thirteen weeks, I walked out of the center feeling a strange familiarity. I had expected to feel different somehow, to see a clear contrast between my eight years of obstetrical care and the care at a birthing center, to feel inspired, as if I had come home. When that didn't happen, I muddled through my feelings for a few weeks until the lights came on: I had to come home to feel like I had come home. The birthing center experience was the stepping stone I needed to see that if I could get past my limited cultural experience, what was really missing was home.

The search was on for the right caregiver to bring our baby into this world in our house. I went with a friend to a prenatal visit with her certified professional midwife (CPM) and was instantly inspired. I left her office feeling a sense of personal responsibility for myself, my health, my baby, and my delivery. From that day forward, I was motivated to eat, sleep, drink, think, and dream toward one goal: a healthy, successful childbirth at home.

I decided to do an experiment and try to have a completely natural pregnancy and childbirth experience. The refrigerator and pantry were transformed; the medicine cabinet gathered dust; and I became a student of pregnancy, childbirth, and nutrition. I traded running for swimming, Tylenol for teas, and Tums for homeopathic remedies. I knew that if I couldn't navigate my way through a headache without popping a pill, there was no way I could face the challenge and joy of natural childbirth. I saw my first birth through allopathic eyes. In my second birth I would leave the well-trodden highways to find find the ancient path of homeopathy.

Yoga introduced me to squats. The health food store yielded a liquid iron supplement that kept me from being anemic. When my legs cramped and my nerves frayed, my midwife directed me to a tasty little calcium liquid supplement. I ate papaya extract for heartburn. I drank three liters of water a day. I slept on my side with the proper alignment of pillows for support. I breastfed my toddler, and my belly grew. I got tired and cranky and hot in the summer heat, but still I grew. I gave up walking in the heat for swimming in the cool water. My close relationship with God helped me navigate a group B streptococcus (GBS) scare. Prayer, pulsatilla, and pelvic tilts turned our baby from breech to head down in the last two weeks of my pregnancy. My one weakness was ice cream, and I ate several pints of peanut butter and chocolate my last few weeks. I grew; the baby grew. My due season drew near.

After the last of my due dates passed—a range of fifteen days— I waited. I walked and waited. I climbed stairs in hopes of generating some action, and waited. My house was clean, my room was ready, the supplies were set up, the books had been read, the class had been taken, the birth plan written, the team assembled, and we waited.

After forty weeks of gestation, my midwife said, "You're going to have this baby next week, so relax." I went home and stopped waiting. I went on with my life, played with my toddler, enjoyed the last of the pregnancy clothes that still fit me, and swam in my string bikini in the backyard pool. My bodaciously round belly protruded past the yellow and gold triangles of my bikini top, and I basked in its glow. I went to bed that night with a name picked out and a sense of peace.

The next morning I awoke early, about three AM, with some mild contractions. I went back to sleep and woke up off and on for the next two hours with contractions. About five in the morning, I began to time them. Ten minutes. Then seven minutes. Soon each rush came five minutes after the last.

We got up, ate breakfast, and played with our daughter. I called the midwife. We talked for a moment, and she went off to feed her farm animals—(she lived on a farm two hours away)—saying to call her if anything got longer, stronger, or closer together.

I went to finish some laundry as my husband and Blythe played together in the living room. Soon we both needed him. She wanted him to play with her; I needed him right by my side for contractions. I leaned over the back of our futon in my bathrobe and said, "Get some help here quick!"

We called my dad to watch Blythe. We called and left a message for our doula friend Heather to come help us get settled in at home. (She took her time coming over; she thought we were in for a long haul.) The midwife was still at her house when we called a second time.

"You better come; I think it's time," Joel said, and I moaned in the background.

"Is that Courtney?!" Ana asked.

"Yes."

"I'll be right there!" She hung up the phone and raced to her car.

As she sped through country roads and city traffic to get to my house, her apprentice arrived and checked my cervix: three centimeters. Phone calls were made so everyone could stop and take a breath. The midwife stopped speeding; the family members gathered in the other room and got settled in for the day.

I began to shed my clothes, any outside thoughts, and any lingering fears in preparation for birth. I walked around my room, enjoying the "push-up" orange color that Joel had painted it just weeks before. I moved to and fro, from my room to the bathroom, squatting, sitting on the toilet, lying on the bed, moaning, resting, laughing, relaxing, then getting a little annoyed when the midwives started chatting amongst themselves or when the phone rang or if my husband was unavailable for a contraction.

It was Friday morning, I was naked, the sun was shining, and it was a great day to have a baby. I wanted to be the center of the universe.

The midwives were concerned that the baby was not putting enough pressure on my cervix for it to dilate effectively, so they sent us on a walk. The walk. It took me several moments to realize that I had to get dressed to go on this walk and that my husband and I were supposed to tootle around my neighborhood until something started to happen. "Twenty contractions," they said. "Don't come back until after twenty contractions, and by the way, walk through every third contraction; you can squat for the rest." Sure, yeah, whatever; no problem. Heather followed us outside to take a picture. It was a rather warm July day but not as warm as I had expected a July day to be. Heather decided to join us, and the walk began.

The first few contractions were intense but manageable. I walked through a few of them and sensed the power of birth swelling up around me. We chatted a little, neighborhood dogs barked, and people stared as they drove by.

By the time we got to the furthest point from my house, I began to think that this walk might not have been such a good idea. We turned the corner of the block to head home, but my little house seemed very far away. I was no longer walking beside my doula and my partner: I was one with them as I interlocked my arms with theirs. I wanted to lie down in the grass after each contraction; my uterus seemed erect and huge; sweat began to trickle down my back.

I squatted at the last corner and felt something pop. I thought that I had messed my pants because my pants felt filthy. It turned out to be bloody show. I was embarrassed but only for a second. All I could think about was getting back to my house and into the shower to clean my self up and then soak in a hot tub.

I fixed my eyes on my station wagon which sat black and gleaming in my driveway under the now blazing Texas sun. It seemed so far away. I could barely walk. My support team was practically dragging me down the street, encouraging me, praising my efforts. I tried to continue walking through every third contraction but found it nearly impossible. I began to speak to the baby: "Peace baby; come down; pressure is good; pressure means baby; peace." A neighbor came out of her house and asked if we needed her to call for some help. No, we said; we're fine, just having a home birth, but thanks.

After what seemed like an eternity, we made it to my driveway. A second apprentice had arrived, and she was going out to her car to get something. She stopped us in the driveway.

"Did you finish twenty contractions?"

"No, but I'm done. No more; I'm going inside."

"I don't know," she said kindly, "She might make you finish all twenty."

"No. I'm finished. I need to get in the bathtub."

At that moment I squatted down in the driveway and my water broke, nice and clear, with a thick, bloody mucus plug right in the middle.

"Uh, okay," the apprentice said, "You can go inside now," and ran in ahead of us.

The midwife met us at the door. It had been forty minutes from the time we had left to the time we were back standing at the door. At the beginning of the walk, I was at three centimeters dilation. When we met the midwife at the door, I was squatting and starting to push.

"Stop pushing. Stop pushing! You don't want to have the baby on the porch, do you?!"

All I could think about was getting to that shower and then into the tub. The family members who had gathered were settling in for a long day's labor and had been thinking about lunch were now scurrying around, fulfilling the midwife's orders. "You, go turn off the air conditioner." "You, get the rags out of the Crock-Pot." "Someone take Blythe." "What's the fastest way to the bedroom?"

On the way to the bedroom we went though my bathroom, and I saw my beloved bathtub at last. "Can't I just get into the tub for a second, just for a second?"

"No. The baby is coming. We need to get to the bed so I can check your cervix."

"What about the shower? Just a quick shower. I think I pooped …"

I remember stepping out of my shorts, seeing blood, and realizing that I had not messed my pants after all. I don't recall how I got free from my white tank top. The world was flashing by in a blur; it seemed like there were lots of people around me, yet I couldn't tell you who they were.

My uterus contracted and the baby barreled through my vagina. The midwives gathered around and checked my cervix: only seven centimeters. *Seven centimeters; don't push!* They checked again: seven centimeters, but very "buttery" (midwife-speak for soft).

It was at this point that I left the bed and went outside my bedroom window and up onto the telephone wire in my backyard, where a bird sat perched watching the festivities. I remember thinking, "Why can't I just go out there for a minute with that bird; I think I will …"

Suddenly I was face to face with my midwife again, her blue eyes piercing, her calm voice commanding: "Courtney, come back to this bed; we are having a baby." Joel kept me from rolling off the bed completely. I caught a glimpse of my mom, who was looking on, her face mixed with worry and excitement. I could hear my dad playing the guitar in the next room. My sister Allison stood nearby, snapping photos. I locked eyes with the midwife and said, "Tell me what to do."

"Push. Now stop. Breathe: Huh Huh Huh Huh HUH. HUH HUH! Okay, now push a little more." They were reaching in to move that last lip of cervix out of the way of my baby's fast-emerging head. When there was no cervix left, I was given the go-ahead to push, but there was no longer any pushing effort on my part, as the baby made her way out with or without anyone's say-so. I felt nothing except for everything, and then everything went numb. I did not tear, only a skid mark with no repair needed, but I don't know that I would have been aware of it if I had.

Expert hands were all around me, hands on my uterus, hands at the birth canal, hands on my perineum. They squeezed here and tugged there. Something was happening; they were working hard, their voices were calm but firm. I never did hear anyone utter the phrase "shoulder dystocia" but later heard the midwife say to her apprentice, "Have you ever seen shoulders that stuck?"

"No, I don't think so," was her reply.

One more push and out she came. I knew she was a girl. Somehow in the rush of the moment I caught a flash of her tiny vagina, and I knew her name immediately: Fiona. Her creamy skin and pink lips wrapped a blanket around my heart that sent me into ecstasy. A girl, my baby girl, born at home, in my bed, in the orange room that we had painted for her. Here she was safe and sound, pink and crying just enough to let us know that she had a voice.

Everything else after that was a blur, the bed, the hot bath, the fruit and cheese brought to my bedside—all seemed peripheral compared to Fiona, snuggling in my arms, nursing at my breast, trusting in my presence.

There hadn't been any time to play CDs or light candles; the birthing ball was inflated and ready but sat unused in the corner. Phone calls had been made to tell people I was in labor, and no one expected the second call to be, "It's a girl! Fiona Erin Wyrtzen is already here!" but she was: nine pounds even; twenty-one inches long; making her entrance like a bursting ray of light, leaving only a tiny skid and empty womb in her wake.

The heart-shaped placenta slipped out several minutes later. I was barely aware of this last stage of labor as I nuzzled and nursed our precious arrival. Fiona never left my sight. She was cleaned and weighed and cuddled all at my bedside with family and friends looking on.

Fiona was born on a Friday morning, delivered by midwives, attended by a caring doula and a loving family close by. We as a family were spoiled forever by the inspiration and empowerment discovered in a baby's birth at home.

⚭

EMMA HUTCHINSON AND JONATHAN SCHUT'S
BIRTH STORY

THANK GOODNESS FOR memory. It was a peaceful birth, and I am blessed with images of that night and day when our family was born gently into being. Over the course of my pregnancy, I went from feeling terrified and overwhelmed by the idea that my body would have to endure birth, to feeling curious and excited about the time that my body and spirit, together with the spirit and body of the baby inside me, would experience this miracle, this rite of passage. Dominant images of chaotic, painful and sterile births slowly receded, and in their place arose images of strong, powerful women, quiet women, loud women, dancing women, squatting women, kneeling women; women alone, with their partners, with their children, with other women; women in water, in the ocean, by a river—all fully capable of giving birth in their own beautiful ways.

This shift happened gradually. I read positive birth stories in Ina May Gaskin's *Spiritual Midwifery* and in *Birth Issues* magazine. I talked with many wonderful women about their birth experiences. My partner Jonathan and I are blessed with friends and family members who believe in the power of women to give birth. Throughout the pregnancy, we did some shamanic journeying, which helped us connect with the baby and work through any fears we might have. We took a prenatal class that focused a great deal on spiritual preparation for birth. I wasn't sure how I would handle labor, but by the time nine months passed, I felt excited and nervous knowing that my body and spirit and my baby's body and spirit would soon experience a miracle together.

My contractions started on Friday night around eight o'clock. They felt a lot like menstrual cramps, which had also woken me up the night before but had gone away during the day. I went straight to bed, wanting to get a good night's sleep in case this was labor. I wasn't hanging on to the idea that it was; it might have been just the brownies I ate after supper that night. But midnight came, and I wasn't able to get to sleep through these cramps. So I drew a bath, got in, and felt better right away.

At around three in the morning, I woke Jonathan up. "Jonathan, look, I have bloody show! I think I'm actually in labor!" He got up, and we danced through the contractions, which were quite regular. It felt nice to hang on to Jonathan. We would sway and tone through the contractions. They felt pretty strong, and it helped to move and sing through them.

The contractions were coming pretty regularly, about every minute. As seven o'clock in the morning came, we headed into the birth clinic in town. I wasn't sure how the forty-minute drive would be. I watched the sun slowly rising behind us and the yellow straw rising through the snowy fields, giving me strength through the contractions.

Unfortunately, when we got to the center, I had to check in and sign some forms. This slowed my contractions almost to a stop. The nurse insisted I be hooked up to a monitor and, being in no mood to argue, I complied. This was uncomfortable and I think unnecessary.

Afterward Jonathan and I tried to nap, and my contractions picked up again. It was around this time that we met our nurse, Ava, who would support us for the next ten hours. Shortly afterward Noreen, our midwife, arrived. I felt happy to meet Ava and know she would be one of our supporters because I trusted her to respect whatever way we chose to work through labor.

Contractions progressed slowly through the day. Jonathan and I went for a couple of walks. The first walk was beautiful. The sun was a perfect circle in the hazy sky, and I imagined its rays coming down and helping the muscles in my uterus pull up and open my cervix. The moon was a waning half moon. We walked slowly through the contractions. The second walk was not so pleasant. I felt a lot of pressure on my bowels, and we turned back soon after we started. I jumped into the kiddie pool right away, where I stayed, warm, for the rest of the time. When the contractions became more intense, Jonathan played the didgeridoo, an Australian aboriginal instrument with a low, rich drone, while I toned or chanted. There were colorful sea creatures decorating the inside and outside walls of the kiddie pool, and I remember letting myself drift into a fantasy undersea world.

Night came, the sun went down, and Jonathan lit some candles. I was nine centimeters dilated, and Ava told me that the time was nearing when I would push our baby out. She said that the pushing often takes some time. This was the first time during the labor that I lost my serenity. I became afraid, realizing that there was no going back. Interestingly, this is the part of labor I'd seen so many times on film: the hard labor, the actual birth of the baby. Those images took me out of my body a bit, I think, and into my mind's eye. I was panicking, shaking, and expressing my fear.

This is when Ava and Noreen stepped up. They gave me all their love and support, and I gave them all my trust in return. Jonathan hopped into the pool with me, but I asked him to let me have some space. We had been such a great team all day, but now I needed the presence and support of these wise women. I trusted them because I knew they'd each given birth to their own babies and had also witnessed many births. It gave me strength to have them there and to know this. They talked me through the rest of labor, past my feelings of despair and into a more serene and confident state.

When the pushing came, Noreen said, "You have had such a gentle labor so far, and you can continue to have a gentle birth. Just push down, down, down." Ava said, "Your body knows how to do this. Just open up and let your baby out." I can't express enough how important it was to have these two women support me through this final stage. Noreen said, "Good. That was a good strong push. Now I bet if you reach down, you'll feel your baby."

This is when I knew it wouldn't be much longer. The great mystery was upon us; I was opening up to a new world. I can't describe the feeling of being in this powerful stage of transition, between two worlds; we were fully in this moment.

One more strong push and the child's head popped out. I don't remember what Jonathan said, but whatever it was, it felt good. "Emma, you're doing amazing. He's so beautiful." The room was radiating; we were radiating, ready for our baby. At this point the fear was gone. I knew that the hardest part was over and that it would take just one more push. I waited, holding Noreen's hand, for that last contraction that would give birth to our family. Aya's head just floated in the water, waiting. It seemed like a significant moment. And then it came. I pushed his body the rest of the way out, into the water, and into Jonathan's waiting hands. I couldn't believe it. "I did it; I can't believe it!"

I spun around to see my babe held, floating in the water, all curled up. He looked so small, and I reached in and pulled him up, feeling his weight in my arms for the first time. Now we were three, our family.

I hardly slept all night, watching our baby, listening to him breathe. The next morning, Jonathan and I named him Aya Cedar Garland Schut.

Claudia Villeneuve's birth story

"Be prepared to lose this baby." Those were the exact words my obstetrician used when I shared with her my desire to have a vaginal birth at home, after having had my first baby by Caesarean section. She said my uterus scar would rupture. Of course I did not believe her.

Six years before, after a normal first pregnancy, I was brimming with health as my due date passed with no sign of labor. My obstetrician booked me for an induction one Wednesday morning, but the induction failed. By Thursday morning I had a beautiful baby boy in my arms, but also a scalpel-sliced uterus.

It took me about six months to realize that I was not happy with the way the birth had been handled, and I began telling myself how needless that caesarean had been. Maureen, a midwife I met, told me that postponing that realization protected me from suffering while the birth was recent. It was emotional detachment. Neither the baby nor I were ever in any danger or distress; the caesarean was just done because the labor was not progressing, which I blame on the induction and other interventions.

My life continued as it was until the day I found out I was pregnant again. With the new pregnancy my survival instincts kicked in and I thought: "I am not having another caesarean. No way, José." Thus began my search for what I later found out was called a VBAC, for vaginal birth after caesarean.

The frightful and fateful meeting with the obstetrician, who had performed the first caesarean and who told me to be prepared to lose this baby, only confirmed my decision to give birth to my second child at home rather than the hospital. Hospitals have scalpels, and my instincts screamed at me to have my baby as far away from a scalpel as possible. That is when I began attending meetings at the local VBAC association and at the Association for Safe Alternatives in Childbirth. I also began reading *Birth Issues* magazine and books like *The VBAC Handbook*.

My husband Norm was not sold on the idea of home birth right away. In fact, he asked me to promise to have a hospital birth. In the following weeks, every time we talked about the location for the birth, I ended up in tears because I felt he did not understand me. I told him I was reluctant to "give up" my body to the medical establishment that had failed me. Eventually, Norm reconsidered and supported my choices but had only one demand: "If you are getting a mid-wife, then get the best one in the city." This proved to be an easy demand to meet.

Noreen was my first and only interview for a midwife. She seemed convinced that I could give birth at home just fine, and that a uterine rupture due to the caesarean scar was not an issue. She even specialized in water births, an idea that I had fallen in love with by then. Noreen commented on my sunny disposition and my radiant self-confidence. She said I would do very well. Finally I had a supporter. The fact that she had attended over two thousand births helped to seal the deal with my husband. Now I was ready to play the game.

I told absolutely everyone I knew that I was having a home birth to avoid a caesarean and give the baby a gentle birth. Every time I explained my arguments against caesareans, they became more daring. My boldest one was when my dentist asked what was wrong with caesareans, and I said: "It is like deciding to slice open the cheek to extract a tooth instead of simply opening your mouth. It does not make sense." And that is how I made it through the pregnancy: envisioning this dream of a vaginal birth after caesarean coming true. My attitude was totally positive; the execution was still to come.

The pain, oh the pain. One week after I finished working at my engineering job, early labor began. The due date was still another week away. It caught me by surprise. That night I stayed up late preparing a poster chock-full of motivational phrases that I had began collecting months before from the birth books and magazines I had read. These were some of my favorites:

"I have got the will of a sorceress."

"Wear something pretty, eat something healthy, smile—you are having a baby today."

"Smile through your perineum."

"When uninterrupted, ninety-five percent of births are uneventful."

"I did not have one pain I did not love."

But my absolute favorite motivational phrase was: "A healthy baby is the ice cream, the VBAC is the hot fudge, a home birth is the whipped cream, and the water birth is the cherry on top." I wanted my ice cream baby, with everything on top.

The next day I still had early labor and managed to attend my baby shower. That evening the contractions intensified and I began to realize the magnitude of the pain. Tears started to roll. We called Noreen and she sent her assistant Marlo to provide support while she finished with another birth at the local birthing clinic.

I changed positions many times to try to deal with the pain in my back and lower abdomen. Pretty soon I began to ask for the pool, since all I wanted was to get in the water. Noreen came and set up the pool at around seven on the morning of April seventh. Serious labor began, but the baby turned out to be still twelve hours away.

Mentally and emotionally I had to let my body work at opening up, but I had never made it to this point of advanced labor before, which caused me to lose my cool. Only Norm's magical hands pressing my aching lower back brought me relief. I remember saying over and over: "Why does it have to hurt so much? This is ridiculous."

My friend Ana came to help us, and she held my hand for hours. She was pregnant too, and her experience with her three previous babies was a definite bonus. Unfortunately, Ana only got to see me at my worst and had to leave before the birth to pick up her children. She missed a miraculous transformation inside me.

I was at six centimeters dilation, four short, when I decided to take charge. I asked my midwife and my husband to leave me completely alone in the pool and to be very quiet. I had to reach the depths of my soul to come to the realization that the pain of the contractions was unstoppable, unless ... I gave birth. Bingo! I had forgotten that the baby was the goal. I then began to pray to God to give me strength. I asked Him to give birth to this baby Himself because I could not do it. At this magical point, I unknowingly surrendered to Mother Nature by transferring the control to God. It worked like a charm. In the quiet of my home, I closed my eyes and stopped my loud moans, which gave way to a peaceful state in which I managed to sleep for two hours in the pool.

The sensation of pushing began to get stronger and stronger. Noreen roused me from my sleep to ask me to change positions in the pool and allow her to check my dilation. I had reached total effacement (thinning of the cervix) but the dilation (opening of the cervix) was at seven centimeters. I could not believe I was so close and yet so far. Noreen manipulated the cervix and, along with my pushing, this helped me reach full dilation. Noreen could see the baby's head and mentioned that it was not too big, bless her.

I hung on to that positive statement and began to push. Norm held me from behind, and I pushed onto his hands. I was so strong that I almost pulled this big man into the pool with me. The baby's head began to slide down, which felt marvelous, way better than the contractions had felt. I visualized the baby's forehead sliding out and then the ears. When the head came out, I stopped and asked for my five-year-old son Nicholas to come and watch. My fifteen-year-old cousin Diana was entertaining him elsewhere in the house. They both came in time to see the baby's body slide out into the water. The contractions stopped immediately and relief washed over me. Noreen scooped the baby out of the water into my arms. It was all over. I had achieved my dream. The integrity of my caesarean scar was never an issue. "When uninterrupted, ninety-five percent of births are uneventful." Boy that is so right.

In the aftermath, we were caught up in the magical moment: I kept staring at this beautiful and serene baby girl with water up to her chin; Norm and my cousin Diana were quietly moved to tears; my son kept saying "the baby is very cute, the baby is very cute"; and Noreen—well, Noreen had more work to do checking the health of both of us. We named our VBAC baby Isabelle Esther. Thank you to all my helpers and supporters. Thank you, Sant Ji, God.

Birthing naturally with a physician

Dawn Freeman

N ATURAL CHILDBIRTH IS loosely defined as labor and delivery without pain medication. It is also birth in which the woman is able to respond to her instincts, those of her body, of the situation, and of the birth, because she is the only one who feels her body's needs. She has educated herself and developed the determination to give birth the way she wants. She has made a birth plan and ensured that the professionals around her are aware of it. She has surrounded herself with support people willing to follow her wishes. She is in control, makes the decisions, and takes responsibility for her choices about the birth, and because the details have been taken care of, she is able to relax and turn her focus inward on her birthing journey.

It was commonly thought that this kind of birth is only possible at home with a midwife, but women now plan and achieve natural birth within the medical system, in a hospital with a general practitioner or obstetrician as the primary caregiver and nurses as support, alongside their own personal labor support team. More physicians are willing to assist women in the goal of natural childbirth, more nurses are skilled in natural techniques to assist labor, and more hospitals are set up to facilitate nonmedicalized labor and delivery; and the more women there are demanding these options, the more open to those options the medical system will become. Hospitals now have "LDR rooms" with labor, delivery, and recovery in the same room; showers and/or tubs for laboring; midwife delivery privileges; and nurses who are also midwives or trained labor assistants. Hospitals also offer the option of "rooming in" (mother and baby stay in the same room), as well as assistance with and encouragement of breastfeeding immediately after the birth.

Of course, many hospitals are not yet completely enlightened, just as many physicians and nurses are unsupportive of the natural way, but it is encouraging that things are changing in response to the ever-increasing demands of women to give birth the way they want.

It is a challenge to give birth naturally within the medical system. In fact, within the medical model, some medical intervention is seen as unavoidable for almost every birth. It sounds disheartening, but don't let this defeat you; instead, let it incite you to become prepared. To get the birth experience you want, you must take responsibility and be your own authority and your own advocate: you must become an informed, determined woman; you must know what kind of birth you want and know your options; you must find an enlightened physician and great labor support to assist you; and you must not let any naysayers stand in your way, either in or out of the hospital.

≈≈∾

Informed and determined

NATURAL BIRTH: what does that mean to you and how do you achieve it? You need answers to these questions. After all, how can you expect your husband or partner, your physician, and eventually the hospital to go along with you if your reply is, "I don't know"?

In order to find answers, or even to know which questions to ask, you need to become informed. There are three ways to do this: talk, listen, and read! Talk to other moms. Most will be more than happy to tell you about their experiences, both good and bad. This is also a good place to start getting names of physicians, ones to contact and ones to avoid. (There is more about this in the section about the enlightened physician.) Find out if there are any natural childbirth groups or associations in your area, and then go to a meeting. This can be a great source of like-minded people willing to share their stories. Even if you do not plan to use a midwife, make an appointment to talk with one. Midwives are storehouses of information and may be able to put you in touch with groups as well as recommend books or classes (and you never know, you might even change your mind!). Don't forget to talk with your husband or partner as well. You need to agree on what you want to happen so you can feel confident he or she will be one hundred percent supportive of your wishes if you are unable to stand up for yourself.

Once you have started asking the questions, be sure to listen to the replies. Not everything you hear is going to be an option for you, but you never know where a gem of advice will come from, so stay open-minded. While you are talking and listening, start reading. There are a lot of books, magazines, and Web sites devoted to childbirth. The library is an excellent source, as are other moms' bookshelves, and once you start finding the books that support your ideas about birth, you can buy copies to keep. Finding the right book in the library was one mother's defining moment, allowing her to challenge many of the ideas she had taken for granted so that she became "empowered" and "enlightened with knowledge." Magazines may contain interesting articles but they are usually limited in detail. Web sites range from terrible to fantastic with every shade in between, but spend the time to dig out the pearls from the sand and you will be well rewarded.

The prenatal class that you will come into contact with later in your pregnancy is another excellent source of both theoretical and hands-on information. Depending on where you live, you may have access to many different kinds of classes. You will want to find one that emphasizes natural birth and teaches techniques to assist in this. It is very important that your labor support person or team attend these classes with you, or if you are hiring someone, that she is up-to-date with specialized or specific techniques. For example, if you decide to use hypnosis during labor, it would be best to hire a doula or labor assistant trained in using hypnosis for birthing.

By now you should be arriving at some decisions about what you do and do not want to happen and what you are and are not willing to try. Your personal birth philosophy is being formed (or born!). Developing your determination is the next step. It is your determination that will help you question prospective physicians, that will aid you in dealing with some people's astonished or incredulous reactions to your plan of a natural birth, and that will enable you to tell the hospital staff a resounding "no!" if they offer you medication for the tenth time after you have said you don't want any. Determined means knowing what you want, knowing how you're going to get it, and making sure that everyone around you knows it too. Determination means sticking to your plan because *you* know what is the best way to give birth for you and your baby. Determination is feeling strong and confident in your knowledge, in your choices, and in your responsibilities for your birth.

∽⊗∼

Birth plan

ONCE YOU HAVE decided on what you do and do not want to happen during your labor and birth, write it all down. This is called a birth plan, and you will be surprised at how effective it can be. At the top of the page, you can write your mission statement: say what you are going to do, not what you might do; "might" leaves the door open to self-doubt and compromise. The rest of the plan is a detailed list; here are the topics you might consider:

- Who will be present at the birth?
- What props do you wish to use (pillows, heating pad, birthing ball, etc.)?
- What do you want your surroundings to be like (dim lights, music, familiar objects, etc.)?
- Do you want freedom from time constraints and nutritional restraints?
- How you feel about using pain medication?
- Do you want intravenous lines and continuous fetal monitoring?
- Do you want freedom to use natural alternatives to speed up labor, including the ability to move around as needed?
- Do you want perineal support and massage during delivery to avoid episiotomy?
- Whom do you wish to cut the cord?
- Do you want the freedom to initiate breastfeeding immediately after birth?
- Do you have instructions about newborn care (rooming in, no bottles or pacifiers, no vitamin K drops, etc.)?

You can have your physician look over and sign this plan. When you are admitted into the hospital, your plan can be shown to the nurses assigned to you, making them aware of your wishes and letting them know exactly how to support your labor. Because you have taken the care and time to write your wishes down (and to get your birth plan signed by your physician), you may find that you are not bothered with certain questions or routines, since the nurses already know what your answers will be. You may also find that some nurses will request to be taken off (or to be put on) your birth, which means that you end up with a nurse who fits in better with your preferred style. After giving birth, one mother discovered that two nurses had declined her case because her birth plan declared her wish to birth naturally, leaving the way open for her to gain a nurse who completely respected that choice and helped her achieve her stated goal.

❦

Labor assistants

Once you know the kind of birth you want, it is time to find your labor support team. The role of labor assistant is a very important one, particularly when the birth takes place in a hospital. Many women use their husband or partner as their labor assistant, while others their mother, other family member, or friend; some women hire a doula or professional labor assistant, and some have all of the above. Whoever you use, these people will be your active assistants. This means that they will follow your birth plan, assist with your strategies, and generally do whatever is necessary to help you achieve your goal of having a natural birth. An active assistant is also your first line of defense against hospital staff members who resist your plan. A labor assistant can also help fill forms, answer questions if you are unable to, make sure your birth plan is known, and make sure that well-meaning nurses don't interrupt your focus any more than necessary. A labor assistant can't make a decision for you, but can ensure that you have the time to make it. See the chapter on doulas for more information.

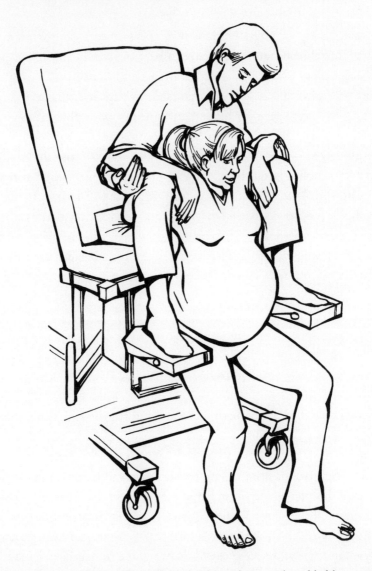

HOSPITAL BEDS can be transformed into birthing chairs with padded knee crutches; removable leg supports; and adjustable length, angle, and locking positions. The woman can use it to birth the baby while sitting upright, or her labor assistant can sit on it and support her in a squatting position. In the supported squat the woman can transfer her weight onto her assistant's knees by leaning on them, plant her feet firmly on the floor, and then relax. Birthing chairs are a far better alternative than using a flat hospital bed for labor and birth. Midwives and enlightened physicians promote upright positions and squatting for labor and delivery because they lead to safer and faster births. Assuming the lithotomy position, lying flat on your back, or even the semi-sitting position actually reduces the pelvic space available for the baby to pass through and can lead to a host of otherwise avoidable obstetrical interventions.

◦⊸◦

The enlightened physician

Your physician should help you feel confident in your ability to have a natural birth and give you ideas on how to achieve this, while at the same time making sure you are informed about what could happen if complications arise. We call this an enlightened physician, and it's more than okay to shop around until you find one. One mother tells of visiting three different health care providers before finding one who would respect and encourage her wishes; another changed physicians when she was twenty-six weeks pregnant, after discovering that her first physician did not understand or agree with her natural birth plan. First, ask other women who have had children who they would or would not recommend. Even ask your own physician for suggestions, especially if you like and respect your general practitioner.

Go to the first appointment armed with questions. A physician who is not willing to spend some extra time answering your questions is probably not going to be supportive of your plans for a natural birth. Some of the things you will wish to know are: the physician's opinion of natural childbirth and willingness to help you achieve it; the physician's opinion of episiotomies and induction, as well as percentage of use of these interventions; and if this is an obstetrician, the physician's rate of caesarean sections. It is not disrespectful or antagonistic to ask questions, and the right physician for you will not mind and will have the answers you want. You may also want to inquire about tests. Physicians do a variety of tests and ultrasounds throughout a pregnancy, but not everyone agrees that they all are necessary. If this is an issue for you, it should be a question for the first visit.

Where a physician delivers can also influence your decision. Some hospitals have a better reputation than others for nursing staff and quality of labor and delivery rooms. You can ask your physician about hospital procedures. Can your support team be with you all the way? Does the hospital require continuous fetal monitoring? Are women encouraged to walk around or required to stay in their rooms and beds? What is the caesarean rate at the hospital, and are there any special procedures in place to discourage unnecessary caesarean deliveries? It might also be interesting to find out, if you can, the hospital's rate of epidural or other medication deliveries and their rate of natural deliveries.

Most physicians work in a practice shared with others, so it is important to find out their actual delivery schedule. Does your physician actually attend each patient's birth, or is your physician on an on-call roster with other doctors? If the latter, you need also to be able to meet and talk with the other physicians in the practice because there is a good chance that one of them will be on call when you go into labor. With any luck, you will find that it is an enlightened practice!

If it is thought that you have a high-risk pregnancy, you will be referred to an obstetrical specialist. You can still be determined to have a natural birth, but again you might need to ask around until you find a physician whose approach is in accordance with your philosophy.

Once you have found the physician of your dreams, don't be afraid to take advantage of this resource. You will only see your physician once a month for most of your pregnancy, so use that time well. Besides asking everyday questions about how you are feeling, take your birth plan to show your doctor. Your physician can help you to prepare a realistic plan, and this is your opportunity to discuss together your labor and birth wishes. Talk over your plans with your physician and maybe even have your labor assistants meet your doctor too. Then tell your body that it must go into labor on whatever day it is that your physician is on call!

~∾~

The hospital

Once you know where your physician delivers, take the tour. This is the best way to learn what kind of hospital it is. (With any luck, your enlightened physician delivers at an enlightened hospital.) The tour will show you the facilities. You may learn whether the hospital offers rooms in which women can both labor and deliver; whether the facilities are comfortable for husbands or partners; and what support the hospital provides for labor. The tour is a great opportunity to ask a nurse about natural birth, birth plans, labor assistants, as well as to inquire which hospital routines are flexible and which are enforced.

You may find out whether there are places and equipment for patients to prepare or store food; or whether the hospital is set up for husbands/partners to sleep overnight. You may find out about postnatal routines (encouragement of immediate breastfeeding, availability of lactation consultants, rooming in with the baby, no bottle feeding at the mother's request, use of vitamin K shot and eye ointment). If you don't like what you see or hear, talk about it with your physician. Maybe he or she also delivers somewhere else. But if not, you might have to decide to find another physician who does. In reality, you will be spending more time when in labor dealing with the hospital and its staff than you might spend with your physician, so it is important that you feel confident that the hospital staff will respect your choices.

A birth center is another birth place option. There are both freestanding birth centers located outside of a hospital, and in-hospital birth centers located near or adjacent to hospital obstetrical units. If this interests you, find out if there are any birthing centers in your area, and check out the National Association of Childbearing Centers (NACC).

Once your labor starts, don't stay still, but stay at home. Most first-time moms go to the hospital far earlier than necessary, and once you are at the hospital, it can be harder to follow your birth plan. In addition, it is a common conditioned response to let people in authority take over, so if your assigned nurse is not supportive of your birth plan, it can feel difficult to override her. Home is more comfortable and relaxed, with better access to snacks, drinks, showers, baths, and other natural interventions. At home there is room to move about without feeling shy or embarrassed. Wait until those contractions are very close together before picking up your bag and leaving, unless of course you feel worried or afraid.

~◌◌~

The nurse

The biggest unknown you will have to face is the nurse assigned to you when you check in to the hospital: you can choose everyone else involved in your pregnancy and birth except this one. Some nurses are well practiced in helping women labor and deliver. Some are even midwives as well as registered nurses and have a wealth of strategies and advice to offer. In the birth stories in this book, one mother mentions how fortunate she was to have a nurse on her case who was also a midwife and how much she valued her calming statements and presence. Another found the nursing staff fabulous: the nurses asked only once if she wanted an epidural, then didn't mention it again when she declined, and told her to do whatever she needed and that they would work around her.

When you meet your nurse, it is important to politely but determinedly communicate your intention to labor and deliver naturally and communicate that you don't want offers of medication every time you wail in pain. This is where your birth plan and labor assistants can help. Have one of your labor assistants show the nurse your birth plan. You will be surprised at how many nurses will respect a woman's planned wishes. A nurse will expect you to comply with external fetal monitoring, internal check for dilation, and blood pressure checks. If you don't want these things, it is your right to say no. This is where it becomes important that you previously researched the hospital policies: if your nurse tries to insist, you can confidently insist back.

Unfortunately, some nurses will not respect your wishes or will think they know better than you what you should do. Be determined and confident when dealing with nurses like that, and make sure your labor support can be determined in the face of authority on your behalf. In one birth story, a woman recounts that she was singing through her contractions, which was not popular with the nurses on the ward, but when a representative was sent to silence her, her husband calmly said that his wife would do whatever she needed to do. It is important to realize, however, that while your husband or partner can give instructions directly to the nurse, your doula or other labor assistants cannot. A doula or labor assistant can run interference to get you more time to make a decision, or can explain things to you in clearer language, but you must communicate your decisions to hospital staff.

Nurses should provide a relaxed, comfortable, supportive atmosphere while at the same time answer your questions and stay alert for any signs of distress. While nurses have experience from attending many births, they do not have absolute authority over your body or your birth and do not have the right to disregard your wishes. Remember, a nurse cannot force you into anything without your consent. If you are extremely unhappy with your nurse, you could try to have your husband or partner ask the hospital if another nurse could take over your case. Now you are determined and informed, you have a birth plan and many strategies to manage your labor, as well as the help of an enthusiastic and active labor assistant and an enlightened physician. How can you fail to have a natural birth? Well, the best-laid plans. . . . Being determined and informed does not guarantee you your ideal birth. Every birth is unique, and sometimes things happen that are out of your control. Your having found and worked with an enlightened physician throughout your pregnancy does not mean that person will be available to catch your baby when the time comes, and knowing that you have the right to refuse standard hospital procedures (if you and your baby are doing fine) does not make it easier to face down hospital staff. But everything you have learned does mean that you can feel satisfied you were prepared and tried your absolute best to birth your baby naturally, even if the end result is not what you planned. With a little bit of luck on the same side as all that good planning, you could become part of a wonderful hospital statistic that I hope will grow and grow, that of women who gave birth to a healthy baby and did so naturally within the medical system.

DAWN FREEMAN originally hails from New Zealand and moved to Canada in 1998. She is a mother of two, both born in a hospital using a general practitioner. Her first birth was full of the interventions that she wished she'd known how to avoid, but through education and determination her second was achieved completely naturally.

＠

DAWN FREEMAN'S BIRTH STORY

AT THE END there was a boy. At the end there was joy and wonder and exhaustion and hunger, so much hunger, both his and mine. At the end, there was a new life in my arms, and he was beautiful and perfect and real. At the beginning of the week there had just been me with the urge to drink red raspberry leaf tea, and now the end and the beginning had happened.

My first child, Gala, had been thirty hours in the hatching, starting with my water breaking before a single contraction had ever been felt and ending with the last six hours involving a whole list of medical interventions I had not wanted. It was a slippery slope: first there was the intravenous line for dehydration, then the pitocin for stalled labor, the epidural, the vacuum (failed), and finally the episiotomy and forceps. At least it ended there and not with a caesarean section.

I did not want a repeat episode, so I told everyone that I was not going near a hospital until I was about to give birth, not even if my water broke first as had happened before. I was sure that if I could labor at home, I would give birth without the need for medical help. I thought about hiring a midwife and having a home birth, but there was just not enough money in our coffers and, besides, unlike a lot of women, I actually like the impersonality of a hospital. Scott would be my main support again, and we had confidence in ourselves. We prepared ourselves by reviewing old techniques and learning new ones to manage the pain of labor naturally.

Just over a week before my given due date, I started having a strong desire for red raspberry leaf tea. I bought some and began drinking two or three cups a day. Four days later, I woke early to strange wetness, and my first thought was despair: my water had broken first again. It wasn't that, but it did turn out to be the beginning of the final show. All day slow, contractions of medium strength spread through me, strong enough to feel but not strong enough to cause me to stop what I was doing. I walked back and forth in the house, since the snow was knee deep outside. I read books to Gala from a squatting position. I drank more red raspberry leaf tea and ate soup and toast. When evening rolled around, things had actually slowed down, and I despaired again that it was just a false alarm. Still, we sent Gala to stay the night at her grandparents in case the contractions picked back up. Trying to be smart and conserve my energy, I went to bed early. Scott, foolishly as it turned out, did not.

It was one in the morning when a sledgehammer in my stomach woke me. Contractions that had been of medium strength were now extra strong, with only a short pause between them. I pressed the heating pad against my back and breathed and moaned and counted and eventually woke Scott up. Soon, lying down was too hard to manage, and we moved into the living room. I paced and squatted, holding on to the arm of the chair. I counted out loud through each contraction until I could speak no longer, and then I counted in my head. I perched on the edge of the couch, leaning back against Scott, with the heating pad between us. I didn't want him to speak to me at all and yelled at him when he forgot. I needed no external distractions to take me away from managing my pain. We spent three hours like this, and then suddenly at the end of a contraction, squatting next to the chair with my head on its arm, I had reached my limit. It was time to go to the hospital. Scott called a cab and then helped me into snow boots and jacket, hat and gloves. It was minus twenty degrees outside, crisp, clear, and lightly snowing.

When we arrived at the hospital, I ignored the wheelchairs and slowly walked to the desk and then to a labor/delivery room. The distraction of the car ride had helped and I was feeling strong and in control again, that is until I had to lie down and have the monitor belt put on me. The worst thing about hospitals is the machinery they always want to use. But everything was fine, so I quickly got rid of it. I thought I wanted to stand and walk again and then realized that I couldn't, so I turned on my side instead, with pillows placed everywhere for support. From this point to the birth was only one hour, and I remember only fleeting images from it: the constant pain (but after one refused offer of morphine the nurse didn't ask me again), the student doctor asking irrelevant questions, the student emergency medical technician whose arm I probably bruised, the relief of my water breaking, and the agony of turning to my back and sitting up to push, my doctor (my *actual* doctor, who was on call that night) coming in right at the end and telling me to save my breath for pushing (I hadn't realized until then that I was screaming the pain out). And then it was done.

Just like the first time, I didn't even hear my doctor say what the baby's gender was. I was too busy lying back and resting. But then my boy was put into my arms, with his eyes wide open, and it was wonderful to meet him at last. He suckled straight away as I delivered the placenta and got one small stitch. Everything went just the way I wanted it to: no interventions, no medication, no drama; it was a straightforward and wonderfully ordinary birth and exactly the way I wanted to start a new life.

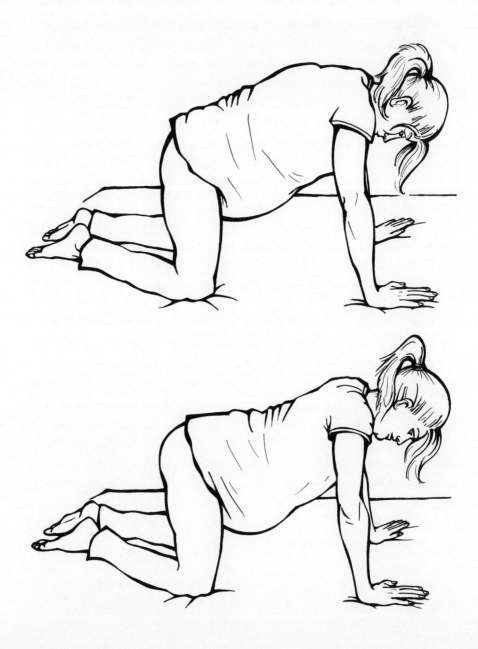

THE ALL-FOURS POSITION is an optimal position throughout pregnancy, labor, and birth. It provides an excellent way to reduce stress on the lower back, which is especially helpful to pregnant women, who have the added weight of the baby, the placenta, and the amniotic fluid to carry around. Doing back arches, known in yoga as cat poses, can aid in proper back alignment during pregnancy, relieving lower back discomforts. During labor the all-fours position allows the baby and the pelvis to float freely in the air as opposed to being constricted by a bed. An all-fours position aids in rotating babies to optimal birth positions, reduces excessive pressure in the perineum that might lead to perineal tears, and relieves back labor pain caused when the baby's head, not the face, is pushing on the woman's spine. When babies are born "sunny-side up," facing the mother's front, usually labor is a little longer and more intense because the baby needs to maneuver more. The all-fours position helps because the mom can rock her body to the rhythm of the contractions and even birth the baby in this position.

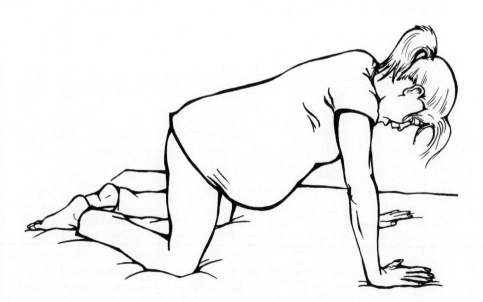

⚭

Karlene and Jim Taylor's birth story

When my husband and I found out we were pregnant with our first child, I realized that we were embarking on a whole new journey. I began to buy books to help me understand all that I would go through in the next nine months. I really enjoyed reading about pregnancy, and I soon figured out that there were many different opinions about the whole process of labor and delivery. I knew one thing for sure: I wanted to have a natural childbirth. I did not want drugs or any unnecessary interventions. I just wanted my body to have a chance to birth a child the way Mother Nature intended.

As I began thinking more about labor and delivery and remembering all the stories I had heard of long, agonizing, painful childbirths, I couldn't help but second-guess myself. Could I really do this? Through a friend, I had heard about a class that used hypnosis to create an easy, fast, and painless childbirth. My husband and I decided to take it. It was one of the best decisions we have ever made in our lives.

We took a class through Hypnobabies <www.hypnobabies.com> with an instructor named Kerry. We attended classes on six Fridays for three hours each. We not only learned about hypnosis in this class, but Kerry also taught about nutrition and how to advocate for oneself in the hospital when it came to making decisions. I learned what was necessary and what is often not when you're dealing with institutional routines. This helped my husband and me feel educated and empowered when we needed to work with the hospital workers to create the safest birthing for our baby.

In preparation for our baby to be born, we listened to hypnosis tapes and CDs, and my husband read hypnosis scripts to me. I also did several exercises to help my body and my baby get ready. Originally I thought the concept of hypnosis would be a little weird. I have never done anything like it before. I soon realized that there was nothing weird about it. It was a discipline that taught me to relax and focus to help my body have this baby just the way it was made to. It seemed like a lot to do at first, but I soon reframed it to be a time to lie down and relax for a half hour each day. I wondered if it was working. I thought: am I really being hypnotized? I soon put all the worrying aside and decided it was working. And it was; I just needed to believe it was.

As my date was approaching, everyone kept asking me how I was feeling. Was I nervous, scared, or worried? I could honestly answer, "No, not at all." I felt confident, ready, and relaxed. The class helped me reach this point.

My date was February eleventh, and on Tuesday morning, January twenty-second, my journey began. I woke up at nine in the morning and felt sort of a pop. I did not know what it was, but I got up because I thought I needed to go to the bathroom, and to my surprise water was running down my leg. I thought: oh, my water broke. I was very calm and poked my head out the bedroom door to tell my husband. He said okay very calmly. We had both decided that we wanted to stay home as long as possible, so I cleaned myself up and went about my regular business. I had no contractions, and I felt fine. I took some time to pack my bag and bake some brownies for the nurses with a "thank you in advance" note. I relaxed in my recliner and just reflected on how my life was about to change. I really did all of this, and it was quite nice.

At about one in the afternoon, I started to feel some small contractions. I wasn't sure if they were real contractions because they didn't feel very strong and I still felt fine. Each time I felt one, I closed my eyes and used my hypnosis techniques. At five PM, Jim and I decided to go to the hospital, mainly because I was concerned about traffic and it seemed like the contractions were getting stronger, but I still felt very relaxed. We called our hypnobirthing instructor, Kerry, because we had asked her to be with us during our childbirth. I checked in at the hospital, and at first the nurses didn't believe that my water had actually broken. I got the feeling that they thought I was going to be there a long time because I seemed so calm. I sat in the big chair right next to the hospital bed and just stayed there, continuing to practice my hypnosis techniques.

The doctor came in and introduced himself. My regular doctor was on vacation. This was at seven thirty PM; I had only been at the hospital for about two hours. I heard him tell the nurses to call him at home when I was further along. He then came over to me to ask a few questions. He told me to tell the nurses when I felt pressure like I had to go to the bathroom. I looked at him and told him that was how I was feeling right then. I kept asking him to stop talking so I could concentrate through a contraction. He noticed that I was doing that often and decided to do a vaginal check before he left. The doctor checked me and he said with his eyes wide, "You are at a nine; this hypnobirthing must really work." I was dilated nine centimeters, and I think everyone at the hospital was very surprised that I seemed so together.

I was feeling the contractions pretty strongly at this point, but it was nothing like I had heard from so many people. During each contraction Jim would read portions of our hypnosis scripts to help me focus and get through them. Kerry showed up and also helped me with my hypnosis techniques. I worked through one push at a time. I vividly remember telling myself to take one push at a time. My hypnosis helped me relax between pushes. I think I would have been tense, anticipating the next push, if I hadn't learned how to relax and let my body do what it needed.

At eleven minutes after ten PM, my beautiful baby boy Conner James Taylor was born. He was eight pounds three ounces and twenty-one and a half inches long. I did it without anything connected to my body, no drugs, and no intravenous line, just my body doing what it knows how to do. I truly believe that my hypnobirthing class prepared me to have a smooth and gentle childbirth. When Conner was coming out, it was an incredible feeling to know that my body was created to have this baby without any interventions, and because I was relaxed and ready, Conner was ready to come. Was it painless? Yes, it was beautiful! Pain would never be the word I would use to describe my experience.

When Conner was ten months old, my husband and I found out we were having another baby. We decided to attend the hypnobirthing classes again. I had all the material, but I wanted us to take the class again to refresh our memories and to help us stay accountable to our daily hypnosis scripts and tapes. I had a little more anxiety with this pregnancy because I had such a great experience with my last and I didn't want my expectations to be too high. I stayed focused and tried to remember the success of the process.

My due date was June twenty-seventh. On July fourth, I was wondering if my little one was interested in ever coming out. I was beginning to get pressured to induce, but I felt very strongly that my little baby would come when it was ready. During the night of July fifth, around three thirty AM, I began to feel light contractions. By six thirty in the morning, I woke up my husband and told him that today was the day, finally. I continued to use my hypnosis techniques while feeding my little guy breakfast and getting ready to go. By seven thirty,

I needed to sit in the recliner and really focus. I put my headphones on and listened to my hypnosis tapes.

At a quarter after eight in the morning, I went to the kitchen sink to throw up. I got nervous and told my husband that we should leave for the hospital because I had heard that people throw up when they are in transition or close to delivering. We got to the hospital at eight forty-five, and I walked into the waiting room. I asked my husband to push me in a wheelchair the rest of the way. The contractions were strong, and I knew I was ready. I was settled in my hospital bed at nine o'clock. The nurse was busy asking questions and working with the monitor. My body began to convulse into a push and I remembered the feeling from when I had Conner. I told my husband Jim that I was close. He relayed the message to the nurse; I think she thought, yeah, right, you are close. She hesitantly decided to do a vaginal exam. I heard her screech and announce that I was dilated ten centimeters and the baby was ready to come.

Needless to say, everybody was scurrying, and they had to call in an emergency delivery doctor because at nine thirty AM, a half hour after I got to the hospital, my beautiful baby girl was born. Emma Elaine Taylor weighed nine pounds, and she was twenty-one inches long. Once again my body was free of an intravenous line. It was a very fast experience. However, I don't think I will wait as long next time. That was a very close call.

Jill Koziey's birth story

SATURDAY, AUGUST SIXTEENTH, six minutes after two in the morning, I am suddenly awake and I cannot figure out why. All at once I simultaneously hear and feel a curious pop, and I realize that my water has just broken. I get out of bed, but within a few seconds, I experience a massive contraction that brings me to my knees, stopping me short on the way to the bathroom. This is really it; I'm in labor! The excitement I feel is almost overwhelming, but I keep it to myself as I shower. No point waking my husband Brent yet, as I could have contractions all night long and at least one of us should get some sleep.

Brent hears me in the shower and immediately suspects what is going on. I suppose it is somewhat obvious, given I am not normally prone to take showers at two in the morning. It's fortunate that Brent has awakened, because once I've finished showering, the contractions begin to come very strongly and are only three minutes apart. Brent phones the birth center at the hospital to tell them that we are on our way and then calls our doula, Ivy, arranging to meet her at the center. Brent also calls my family in Calgary, saying simply, "It's show time!" then quickly hangs up to help me to the car. I smile to myself at the flurry of activity I envision at my sister's house in Calgary as they prepare for the drive up to Edmonton.

As Brent drives the twenty minutes to the birth center, I vocalize with every contraction. I am amazed at the "song" that comes out of me, one long, unwavering note. I am intensely overwhelmed with each contraction, yet a part of me is somehow disengaged, watching and acting as a calming, grounding force.

Upon arriving at the birth center, we discover that both of the birthing rooms are already in use. We are guided to a room in the main area of the hospital, and I immediately strip and don my "birthing nightie." The nightie stays on for all of thirty seconds. Naked is how I need to be, and the primal part of me knows that and acts quickly.

The fact that both of the birthing rooms are already being used means that both of the birthing pools are also taken. Because a water birth was of primary importance to me, we came prepared, bringing with us an inflatable pool exactly like those used at the center. Brent breaks out the unused Mother's Day gift that he had given me for the hot days of summer during my pregnancy and starts to inflate it before quickly returning to my side. I continue my song with each contraction, focusing on Brent's eyes and holding his hands with all of my might. However, it appears that my singing is not very popular with the nurses in the main hospital wing where I am stationed, so a representative is sent to silence me. Brent is quick to react, and evenly tells the nurse that I will do whatever I need to do. The nurse protests once more, and Brent simply returns his focus to me. In silence the nurse retreats to the hall, and I continue with what my body tells me to do.

During this time our doula Ivy arrives and easily slips into Brent's position so he can finish filling the pool. Once it is filled with warm water, I make my way, assisted on both sides by Brent and Ivy, across the room to the pool and gratefully slip in to the warmth that quickly envelops my laboring body. The physical relief is instant, and my vocalizations change themselves to communicate with our baby. "Down, Baby, down!" I say over and over again, with each contraction. I had no idea that my voice could go that low, and despite the pain I find myself feeling in awe of my body and how it is doing exactly what is necessary. It is so liberating to stop thinking and to simply let the natural flow of events take over.

For the next four hours, I remain in the pool on my knees with my head resting on Brent's lap during the short space between contractions. Ivy continuously pours warm water from the pool over my back—an amazing feeling—and takes over for Brent whenever he requires a break to go to the bathroom or to add more hot water to the pool (pumping out the cooler water in the process). Our midwife Joanna visits our room periodically to ensure all is going well, and it is always lovely to feel her there. Throughout my labor Brent responds to my every slight nuance, and I feel safe and supported by him. I am keenly aware of the depth of connection that my husband and I are sharing, and I am so incredibly grateful for his presence.

With each contraction, my message to our baby comes out of my mouth in my newfound deep and primal voice. At one point the obstetrics nurse suggests to me that I save my energy for pushing by breathing instead of vocalizing. Suddenly I am confused. Do I need to conserve my energy? I have never done this before. Will I run out of steam when it comes time to push? I stop my spoken words to my baby and instead focus on my breath. The pain becomes overwhelming, and my confusion intensifies. The sounds coming out of me are now high-pitched. I have lost touch with the grounding force that was within me. Seeing me in this state, Ivy leans over and gently whispers that I should do whatever I need to do. I am grateful for this simple sentence, and I relax my mind and let my body take over once more. When the nurse again makes her suggestion, I ask her to "Stop talking"—pause for contraction—"please," and she respects my wishes. I continue as before, following my body and talking to my baby.

I keep expecting the urge to push to come, and when it doesn't, I finally make a conscious decision that it is time to push. As soon as I begin pushing, the physical urge actually kicks in, and it takes only ten minutes for our baby's head to emerge. Curiously, our baby's little hand comes out next to her head, as though in a gesture of greeting. Our beautiful nine-pound baby daughter, Hannah Lynne Elizabeth, is born, drug free. It is three minutes after eight in the morning, and our lives have been changed—and blessed—forever.

꙾

Sue Robins's birth story

A LETTER TO my baby Aaron, whose name is Hebrew for "enlightened and to sing."

Mama's water broke at six in the morning on Saturday, March twenty-ninth. Water trickled down my leg when I went to the bathroom, and I thought, "What the heck is this?" I managed to hold off waking your daddy until six forty AM. You had decided to arrive two weeks early.

Your daddy and I puttered around the house, finished packing for the hospital, and your daddy made me an egg and toast breakfast. I packed a little index card that said: "You can do this." Those four little words reminded me that I was very determined to have you without any medication and, I hoped, without any interventions.

We stopped at Starbucks for a juice and a scone, and arrived at the hospital around eleven AM. I was hooked up to the monitor in the labor and delivery room. There were no contractions, just mild cramps. I became despondent, thinking that I'd have to be induced, as had happened with Isaac and Ella, your brother and sister. I begged to be let off of the monitor so I could walk around, and even bribed the nurses with a box of donuts.

At twelve thirty PM, I was freed from the machine, and your daddy and I started walking around to try to convince you to start making your way out. I drank lots of water to avoid being hooked up to an intravenous line and peed regularly to avoid a catheter. We walked to the main hospital and got a turkey sandwich for lunch. We walked, walked, walked. I got a blister on my foot from so much walking. The staff transferred me to a different ward: antepartum. We asked for a private room and ended up in a full public ward. Luckily we found an empty room for some peace and privacy, and we walked more and more and more.

My doctor visited at three thirty in the afternoon. He said he'd let me try to deliver on my own before considering induction. I wanted so badly to give birth, the first time in three pregnancies, without being induced. We continued to walk, walk, walk. Contractions finally started around four thirty PM, short, mild ones, close together.

We kept walking and stopped in the chapel at the hospital. I am a lapsed Unitarian, and I do believe in some sort of higher being. I sat in the chapel pew, and I politely asked for a happy and healthy baby. That's it. That's all I wanted.

The contractions started getting longer and harder around eight PM, so we stayed close to the ward. Your sister was born very quickly, and I didn't want to give birth on the floor by the staff parking garage.

Your daddy did a fabulous job of supporting me. He walked and walked with me, rubbed my back, reassured me, and talked me through each contraction. I love him so much. I couldn't have done it without him. He is my ray of sunshine.

The resident came and checked me at ten thirty PM. I was four centimeters and ready to move to a birthing room. By eleven o'clock, things went very fast. Hard contractions were coming every two and a half minutes. I had a lovely nurse named Jenn in the birthing room. I got in the shower, but nothing was helping to alleviate the contractions. Your daddy kept reminding me to breathe and to open up for the baby and that you were coming. That helped me a lot.

There were only little breaks in between contractions. They were starting to pile one on top of another. I suddenly wanted out of the shower immediately. Pressure was starting to build in my pelvis, and I could feel your head. Somehow I managed to move to the bed. Now I was really into things. There were hardly any breaks in between those crazy contractions. I remember thinking: they'd better not get worse that this; oh, yeah, I still have to push! Jenn checked me: nine centimeters! No wonder; I was in transition!

Your pressure was moving from the middle of my pelvis to my back. You were getting close to coming. I was very, very excited. I kept thinking, "Yes, yes, yes, the baby is coming." With your brother and sister I had thought, "No, no, no, make the pain go away." Thinking "yes" made all the difference in the world.

There was a flurry of activity in the birthing room. A resident came in and put on his gown. He said he could hear me at the desk! I guess I was making a racket. I was pushing a bit during the contractions. They got the bed ready, and I knew you were close. My nurse kept saying, "Do what feels good for your body." It felt good to push because it distracted me from the contractions. After about three contractions I started to really push. It felt fabulous because I knew I would meet you soon. I pushed and pushed, and your daddy said your head was out, and whoosh! There you were on my belly.

Your daddy and I cried and cried when we saw how beautiful you were.

My doctor walked in, one minute too late! You came very fast at the end. You weighed six pounds fifteen ounces and were happy and healthy, just as I had asked for in the chapel. I'll never forget the feeling of having you on my belly, just newly born. That was the best feeling in the world.

Afterward, the postpartum nurses kept coming in to check my intravenous line and were surprised to discover that I didn't have one! I was so proud to have given birth without even one intervention and no medication. I could, and did, do it! After giving birth in such a natural and wondrous way, all on my own, I knew that I could do anything.

Fast forward to two weeks later. Despite having nursed two other babies, I had a difficult time nursing Aaron in his first week. He dropped an entire pound in four days. We went on a strict nursing regime, and I took Aaron in to be weighed every week. At his third appointment, he started gaining weight, which was a huge relief.

At the end of that appointment, my doctor took me aside: "Do you remember we talked about prenatal testing?" I had declined the tests, knowing that I would carry my baby no matter the result. When he said that, I knew that Aaron had Down's syndrome. Aaron had no obvious signs of Down's except for a round little face, but somewhere deep in my heart I knew that he had Down's when he was a day old, when I had asked the public health nurse if she saw any signs of Down's in my baby, and she said no. So I filed my suspicion away as I was not ready to deal with this unexpected news quite yet. Upon the return of the genetic test when Aaron was four weeks old, we found out that he indeed has Down's syndrome.

Everybody undergoes an initial shock and grieving period after finding out their baby has special needs. The baby we were expecting was not the baby we got. My own ignorance about Down's and my ego (how could I have anything less than a perfect baby?) had to be reckoned with before complete acceptance of Aaron's diagnosis was forthcoming. Then my husband and I fell deeply and madly in love with our baby. We would not change one thing about him, including his Down's syndrome. If he didn't have Down's, he wouldn't be Aaron. He's a beautiful baby, with a quick warm smile and a delicious giggle. I cannot put into words how much we love him.

We are on an unexpected road with our little man, but we are beginning to see how Aaron has opened up a whole new world for us to discover and enjoy. It gives me great comfort to think about Aaron's gentle birth; I believe that his special introduction to the world was the beginning of the new path on which we are now traveling, a path with a child who will teach us much about life and compassion and acceptance.

I believe that my confidence in parenting Aaron will also draw from my birth experience. If I can birth a baby all on my own, I can also raise my child who has Down's syndrome. It is my job to teach Aaron to be true to his name. He is indeed my enlightened child, and we will teach him to sing as well and as loudly as he possibly can.

Dee Dee Kopchia's birth story

When my husband and I were married, it was the first of many wonderful dates to come as we began our life together. We both absolutely loved children and dreamed about one day having our own family. In the spring of 1998, we found out we were expecting our first baby and were overcome with joy. It was a day we had both anticipated, but now that it was going to be a reality, in some ways it was surreal. It was such a tremendous feeling, knowing that one of our lifelong dreams was going to be fulfilled. It was also an exciting feeling to tell family and friends that we were going to have a baby. Knowing how much we wanted a family, most wondered what took us so long.

Pregnancy was such an enjoyable nine months that I wished it could have been longer. The anticipation of preparing the bedroom and making sure that we had everything ready was so much fun. Even shopping for maternity clothes was fun.

When I became pregnant for the first time, the obstetricians were on strike; therefore, I was referred to a general practitioner who specialized in delivering babies, Dr. W. When I met her, I was very impressed with her concern, patience, openness, and thoroughness and decided that she was the type of doctor that I needed. She had a partner in her practice, and I was guaranteed to have either her or her partner at the birth. This was comforting, knowing that I would not get stuck with a doctor or intern that I had never met before delivering my baby.

I had always wanted a drug-free natural birth and said so right from the start. When you discuss giving birth with people, so many have something negative to say. For example, I was told many times to just ask for the epidural, morphine, or other forms of pain relief. I was asked, "Why would you go through the pain of natural childbirth when drugs are available?" I was bound and determined not to have any drugs whatsoever.

My pregnancy progressed normally and many hands wanted to touch my growing belly. I worked until two weeks before my due date. During the last few weeks of my pregnancy, my blood pressure started to rise, which meant visits to my general practitioner every other day to monitor me more closely. On my due date, my doctor thought it would be best for me to be induced. Although I felt great physically, I reluctantly agreed so as to ensure the safety of both my baby and myself, and we were scheduled in the next day.

The anticipation of knowing that our baby was going to be born the next day was almost worse than waiting for my labor to start naturally. Upon reaching the induction room at the hospital, I was hooked up to the monitor to discover that I was already having contractions, but could not feel them yet. I was induced by gel at three fifteen PM by Dr. H. He informed me that I had a perfect pelvis for delivering a baby, which was oddly flattering. I started feeling contractions within an hour.

One of the nurses on duty came into my room to start an intravenous line. I questioned the reason for this, and she advised me that it was to keep me hydrated and in case of an emergency situation. I indicated that I was drinking and eating plenty and did not want an intravenous line at that point in time. I assured her that I would consent to one only should an emergency arise.

I was able to walk around with my wonderful husband, who was with me every moment. This sped up the labor process, and at about five thirty PM, I was back in bed lying on my right side, which was the only position that was comfortable for me. I was having hard contractions about two minutes apart and lasting thirty seconds. (They felt a lot longer than that!)

Various nurses came in quite frequently, asking me if I wanted an epidural. Each time, I politely but firmly responded "no." A short time later, one nurse came in and asked me to sign a waiver for an epidural. This was quite maddening as I had made it clear that I did not want any pain medication. She responded by suggesting that I should read the waiver and sign it ahead of time because I might not be able to do so later. I felt like telling her to respect my choice and to just leave me alone to deal with pain. Now I can see why first-time moms get pressured into having an epidural or another kind of pain relief.

Focusing on the designs in the curtains throughout labor and thinking that I would soon get to see my baby helped me through the challenge of overcoming the intensity of the contractions. Tightly grasping my husband's hand, I was unintentionally digging my nails into him, leaving nail imprints in his skin. He seemed oblivious to the pain that I was inflicting on him because it seemed to help me cope. He did not say much, but every so often he would quietly and calmly remind me about my nails, although it did not change anything.

At seven thirty PM, my water broke. We were still in the induction room, because the hospital was full and no delivery rooms were available. My doctor joked that it was as if a bus full of expecting women in labor all arrived at the same time. My doctor phoned the maternity ward and said, "Find a room because we are coming." As they put me in a wheelchair, my husband was grabbing the cameras and our bags. Running down the hallway, the nurse told my husband to run ahead and push the elevator button. My challenge was to hold myself up on the arms of the wheelchair, to stop the feeling of sitting on my baby's head.

As we approached the overflow delivery room, we were told that we would have to wait a few moments as it was not quite ready for us. Nurses were frantically wheeling equipment out of the room, which was being used for storage. The walls had three-inch green square tiles and a huge mirror overhead. It reminded me of the ones that you saw in old movies, but at that point I was indifferent to the decor. My doctor had been getting on her scrubs and continued to do so as she ran toward us. She knew this baby was coming fast.

My first urge to push came at 7:32 PM as I was moving from the wheelchair to the delivery room bed. My doctor said it was okay to push. She was very patient and observant, and after the first few contractions the baby's head would almost crown. She monitored the baby's heart rate closely. On the third hard push, it dropped to sixty beats per minute, so she determined that an episiotomy was needed to eliminate any distress to my baby. With the next contraction, my baby's head was out. With no pain medication at all, out beautiful baby girl Brittany was born at 7:47 PM on January twenty-second, weighing seven pounds, two and a half ounces and measuring twenty-one inches long. I was so proud of myself knowing that I could be strong and labor naturally on my own with my loving husband by my side. The doctor laid Brittany on my tummy so that daddy could cut the cord.

The most amazing moment during the birth was when our baby's head first came out. The doctor suctioned her airway, but she was still unable to breathe on her own as her chest was compressed in the birth canal. It was ironic how a baby's head could be in our world, yet the baby was still fully reliant on its umbilical cord connecting it to the mother. Only seconds later the doctor maneuvered her shoulders and the rest of her body out, and she gasped her first breath.

The postpartum experience at the hospital was frustrating because there were frequent changes in staff and variations in knowledge about breastfeeding. I never realized I should nurse as soon as possible after delivery and no one told me to do so. We were so excited and busy taking pictures and video and just admiring our new daughter. After all the hard work coming through the birth canal, babies go into sleep mode after about an hour. It is very difficult to get them to nurse when all they want to do is sleep.

Breastfeeding was a definite struggle for us. I was badly bruised from the delivery and the episiotomy and found it difficult to sit up and get into a comfortable position to nurse. Getting her to "latch on" was an event on its own. She would finally do so after five to fifteen minutes, then suck a few times and fall asleep. The nurses wanted to supplement her breastfeeding with formula, but I refused, deciding in advance that my baby would be nursed and receive all of the best nutrients possible. I was determined to work through this and not give up my goal of breastfeeding my baby. Feedings lasted from forty-five minutes to an hour and a half, but I did not mind. My baby was getting the best start in life. It took about six weeks until breastfeeding became a little easier. Through it all I persevered, even though there were times that my nipples were dry, cracked, raw, and bleeding. The pain seemed overwhelming, but Lansinoh cream was my salvation. Several health nurses came to my home to try to help improve my technique and confidence. In addition, I made several visits to a hospital breastfeeding clinic. My determination paid off, and I successfully breastfed my daughter until she was twenty-six months old. She was and still is a very healthy girl who rarely ever gets sick.

In the spring of 2001, I became pregnant again and was very fortunate to have another great pregnancy. It was a natural decision to stay with the same doctor since she knew that I wanted a natural childbirth with no drugs for pain relief.

This time I went into labor on my own. It was quite a shock when my water broke at home while I was going to the bathroom at one fifty AM. It was two weeks before my due date. There I was at two in the morning, calmly washing and curling my hair to look decent for our trip to the hospital. I woke my husband to let him know that I was in labor, and he wanted to leave immediately. Being in no hurry, I told him that I was going to finish my hair and makeup.

I had arranged for my sister to come over and look after Brittany while we were at the hospital, so I called her to come over, and she arrived within minutes. She helped me pack my bag since I had not planned on having this baby quite this early. Her calmness helped, too, as she was visiting with me and helping me do those last-minute things. My contractions were coming on stronger, and I had to breathe through each one while I was still curling my hair. Brittany woke up with all the excitement, and we took our last pictures and video with mommy and the baby inside.

We called the doctor and left for the hospital at three thirty AM. This was the part that my husband enjoyed, as I think he liked speeding along the nearly deserted streets, although he blamed it on his anxiety. We were put directly into the delivery room at three forty-five AM. A quick examination indicated that I was already three centimeters dilated. My doctor arrived only a few minutes after us, as she expected this to be another quick delivery.

My contractions progressed quite quickly, the intensity of them growing stronger and stronger and spaced only a few minutes apart. Again squeezing my husband's hand, breathing through each contraction, and focusing on objects helped as much as it had with our first. I was very fortunate to have a nurse on duty that night who had previously been a midwife in her hometown. This time the hospital was not busy, so Sue was able to stay by my side the whole time along with my husband. What I valued the most were her calming statements during each hard contraction, getting me to imagine lying on the beach in Hawaii, letting the warming sun shine down, watching the water, and relaxing. It truly gave me a feeling of comfort having her beside me.

At seven AM, I was fully dilated and had my first urge to push. The hard labor had begun but lasted only slightly longer than with our first daughter. Unfortunately, another episiotomy was required. With no pain medication at all our second beautiful baby girl, Paige, was born at 7:32 AM on February seventh, weighing six pounds, four ounces and measuring twenty-one inches long. I had succeeded in having a natural birth again. The doctor laid Paige on my tummy so that daddy could cut the cord.

After a quick cleanup, Paige was given to me and I attempted to breastfeed right away. At only ten minutes old, she "latched on" beautifully and sucked for minutes. I was so proud of her and of myself. The difference was the confidence and knowledge that I had garnered with my first daughter. There was no hesitation, which led to immediate success. Breastfeeding continued to go well, and I am still breastfeeding Paige at the age of twenty-four months. She is also a very happy and healthy girl. What I learned with breastfeeding is that I succeeded the first time with determination but the second time with confidence.

⟨⟩

Corinne Hepher's birth story

Wednesday, August seventh, journal entry

"Rob doesn't think it will be two weeks until I labor. He said he's seen changes in me even in the last week. I'm bigger, more awkward and cumbersome, more irritable about dirt, people, and my space. Yeah, sometimes I'm quite impatient. Sometimes I think, "I need more time." Tomorrow is the official due date. I think there's still more time."

Saturday, August ninth, seven am

"Oh, the most frustrating thing about being pregnant, besides being fat and heavy, is having to go to the washroom all the time. I'm trying to stay positive and patient, trying to tell myself the best things about being over nine months pregnant: the baby kicking—I can almost feel a foot or a knee."

I had been having many dreams about meeting this baby and was dying of curiosity, wondering if baby was a boy or girl.

"I do like my belly. It's large, round, and firm. Another good thing is anticipating when this will all be over. Sometimes I wonder, will I ever not be pregnant? Have I ever been nonpregnant? Even Rob forgets that I won't have this belly forever. He says he'll miss it. Yet he can't wait to meet "ba'ee" and hold him or her. Me too. But I'm also thinking about what I have to go through to get there and then the soreness and tiredness afterward. Then I think I should just be grateful for where I'm at now and try to be patient. Life is easy now. I can still pick up and go where I want and when. Aside from the physical limitations, life hasn't changed drastically yet. Well, that's mostly true. I think I even prayed yesterday that I would go into labor. But this baby can come two weeks after my due date, which would be on the twenty-fourth, and that would be perfectly normal. My latest guess is the eighteenth. Shouldn't the due date be the day the baby is ready to come out?"

SATURDAY AFTERNOON

Rob and I were in the mall, cashing in some of my stored-up gift money at The Body Shop. The craziest storm I've ever seen broke out, and we watched it with all of the other people in the mall. I was in fearful awe as the trees across the street disappeared from view and rain and hail accumulated on the ground, even rising above the curb, spilling onto the boulevard. All I felt was sheer terror. It was totally sublime. All day I had been feeling Braxton Hicks contractions, painless tightening of the uterus.

SATURDAY, AUGUST NINTH, CONTINUED

"Rob's been awesome. He does far more work around the house than I do ... I'm so tired, I can hardly move ... I've been feeling some minor pains. I just hope it's my cervix dilating and not a bladder infection—I just want it to be productive pain."

That evening Rob asked me to cut his hair. We got a phone message from friends who said they had prayed for us, prayed that my labor would go well and that everything would happen as I hoped it would. As I was cutting Rob's hair, I started to get grossed out by it all, and I started crying. I was disgusted with the hair and our messy house, the baseboards in particular. Everything was grossing me out, and I felt so irritable. Rob gave me this funny look like "What is wrong with you?" but he didn't say anything. He probably knew I would just tear his head off with my teeth if he even mentioned the obsessive nesting and general state of being pissed-off that precedes labor, signs that we were both aware of but didn't discuss because I didn't want to get my hopes up. In the weeks before the due date, I got frustrated if he gasped, "Are you feeling any contractions?" So we agreed not to get too excited about it. Maybe that's why we were caught in a state of denial when the real thing start to happen.

At around midnight, I was constantly going to the washroom and just couldn't get comfortable and couldn't sleep. I was keeping Rob up with all my stirrings. At one point I just gave up and decided that I would stay on the toilet all night. I might as well because as soon as I'd get up, thinking I was done, I'd have to go again. I felt pressure on my bladder. I started to get worried and thought I might have a bladder infection. I was worried that it might hurt the baby somehow if I didn't get it treated.

So I called the hospital's labor and delivery ward at one AM and told them my symptoms. I told the nurse about the pain. "Well, pain is not normal," she said. What is that supposed to mean, I wondered. The nurse said, "Sounds like you have a bladder infection. Why don't you just come on down to emergency, and we'll take a urine sample and hook you up to the electronic fetal monitor." I wondered why they'd have to hook me up to the monitor. I asked her if they would do any vaginal exams because I didn't want to go through that, and she said in a cheeky tone, "Well, not if you're not having contractions." I hung up the phone and didn't know what to do. I wanted to see a doctor because I felt that something was up.

At four AM Rob said, "Why don't we just start timing these things you're feeling, just in case, and then decide whether or not to go?" So we did, and sure enough, the sensations would start, last for three minutes, and then go away again. They carried on and were five minutes, ten minutes apart, back to five minutes, so at 5:21 AM, I wrote in my journal:

"It feels good to move around when the pain comes on. . . . we prayed for wisdom—to know if we should stay or go . . . to discern what is really happening."

A lot of worry subsided after we timed the sensations I was having, yet I was in denial at this point. I didn't want to get my hopes up, but I was so excited to be in labor. Rob said, "I've read about so many women who go into labor at around four AM, something about the levels of the hormone oxytocin that are present at that time."

I was no longer in denial: "So, I'm in labor. I no longer believe this is a bladder infection but rather contractions. Rob feels incredibly peaceful about it. I guessed August eleventh a long time ago, but I never wrote it down. Rob had guessed August twelfth."

I had a hot bath and was experimenting with relaxation and deep breathing to see if they took the pain away. It did subside. The sun came up, and suddenly it was Sunday.

"This is great. Before it was so intense. I wasn't sure how I would make it. But now I feel so relaxed, like in a dreamy state. I feel the natural painkillers pulsing through me. It is so spiritual. I thank God for being in charge, for getting things started. What comforts me is the verse about 'those who trust in God will never be put to shame.'"

"It's so good Rob's off from work. It's not too hot, and I loved the early morning darkness and stillness. We lit candles and had music playing. I told Rob I wanted to build a cocoon around us, to close off the outside world and focus inward. I didn't want anyone to know I was in labor because I wanted to stay calm, not deal with exciting energy or the pressure of having to get this baby out. We went for a walk in the fresh, cool air and sunshine. It was so wonderful. I brought two combs with me to jab into my palms when the pains came on; this helped."

The contractions were picking up, and I didn't want to leave home except to go for a walk. It was peaceful with just the two of us. We were in a rhythm together. When the contractions came on, he would press into my back or rub my back and it was really nice. It was like he was right there with me, going through the experience too. Now that I look back, it might be the last time we'd really be alone until our birdlings leave the nest. It could be twenty years or more. I should have enjoyed that time more.

My friend Mary came over at around three PM. I had met her just a couple of months ago, and she had had two unassisted home births. She just stayed home and birthed naturally. I had never heard anyone describe birth as ecstatic before. She described the sheer power she felt during and after the birth. My dream was to have a birth like hers. I thought that since she had given birth before, she might know what to look for in case anything was out of the ordinary. We had registered at the hospital earlier just in case we ended up there. Well, things started to change when Mary arrived. My contractions suddenly got more intense.

We started to get the tarps and sheets ready, preparing for the baby. My contractions were getting very intense. After four hours of trying hot baths, rocking, breathing, and Mary's visualization techniques, I started to get discouraged. I was tired and hadn't had much to eat. I tried to eat but felt I couldn't. Mary was trying to encourage me by saying, "I wouldn't be surprised if this baby is born before eight PM." Well, eight o'clock came around, and I didn't feel like things were getting anywhere.

Rob and Mary both kept saying I was doing awesome, but I found it hard to believe. I had been saying, "I just want drugs, and I want to go to the hospital." I said this for a long time. I just felt like I couldn't take it anymore. I was tired; I felt weak and devastated. I just couldn't imagine going on for any longer, and I wanted to quit. Funny how nature takes your body and says, "You're going to keep going whether you want to stop or not." Yet the idea of having to push for possibly two hours when I was so tired was beyond me. I didn't feel like I had control of the contractions anymore. What helped was that when the intensity came on, I would grab Rob and Mary's hands and bear all of my weight on them while leaning over.

Contractions, in my experience, can only be described as being possessed by a tornado and a hurricane while having a wrecking ball hit you in the stomach as you convulse in a seizure. And I swear no one can understand what it's like without going through it, this amazing process of bringing a new life into the world. All I could say at the time was, "God, please help me." I swore I would never go through this again. All I could think of was all the women who for millions of years before me had gone through this and all of the women in the world who had labored recently and the universal connection I felt to each one. They had lived to talk about it. "Why, why, why would anyone in their right mind ever do this?" I wondered. This is just insane, excruciating pain! I swore I wouldn't do it again.

Anyway, eight PM came and went, and I felt like I was in a hurry. I was worried that I was taking too much of Mary's time, and I had my mind set on the hospital and any kind of drug I could get my hands on. Mary warned me that if I got there and was ten centimeters dilated, they might not give me anything and then I'd have to deliver naturally anyway. For a long time, I wavered back and forth about whether to go to the hospital or to stay home. Rob asked me just to make a decision: either stay home or go to the hospital. He was getting worried and wanted me to decide one way or the other.

At around nine thirty, I was determined to go to the hospital and get some pain relief. At that point, the only reason I was staying home was to please Mary, and I felt like that wasn't a good enough reason. At that moment, I gave up on my dreams of a home birth and surrendered to an institutional birth. I apologized and said, "I'm sorry. I really wanted a home birth, but this is too much, and I can't handle it anymore." I told Rob and Mary that I wasn't going to be anyone's hero, and I just wanted something to help me get through this. It was a bad trip, a roller coaster ride from hell, and I wanted to get off.

We got to the hospital, and I told the hospital staff that I wanted anything they could give me. I was six centimeters dilated, and the anesthesiologist was in the operating room and wouldn't be back for an hour. Focusing on the epidural was all I could do to get me through. They gave me morphine, but I didn't notice it in the least. Finally two hours later I was eight to nine centimeters dilated, and the nurse said in a cheery voice, "You're so close; you might even birth naturally before the anesthesiologist has a chance to get here." I thought, "God, no! Give me drugs now!" This was just the opposite of my birth plan. I said no drugs, no this, no that, no interventions whatsoever. Well, things changed when I was actually in labor.

At about eleven PM, the anesthesiologist arrived. Rob said, "Are you sure you want to do this?" I said, "Yes, I'm sure." Although I had been anti-drug and anti-intervention, I was at the point that if they had given me a caesarean section, I would have been happy just to get that baby out of me and stop that nightmare.

Rob thought the big needle was scary. I didn't even feel it; I was eager for pain relief. The pain started to fade away. It was like there were angels in the room and I was transported out of my body and into the heavens. I saw this woman who looked like she'd been run over by a steam train, lying on a birthing bed, talking to her tired and dopey husband, who was fixated on the fetal monitor.

At around eleven thirty PM, after almost twenty-four hours of contractions, Rob said, "You look like you've just been in a car accident" and then he took a picture. I had an oxygen mask on and all kinds of tubes and wires coming and going all over me. With the epidural I didn't feel anything. I finally relaxed but not entirely. Rob kept looking at the monitor, and it was making all these bleeping noises. I was scared that something might happen to the baby. The nurses were also fixated on the monitor. I focused on Rob because I was too scared to look at the monitor. Even though I had wanted the drugs to completely end this all for me, I was still dreading what lay ahead: the pushing. I had to face it. I had given up and felt that I didn't care if someone were to cut this baby out of me. I desperately wanted it to be all over with.

The atmosphere in the room was strangely peaceful. It was dark and quiet, the lights were low, and people were speaking with hushed voices or were silent. I was glad about that. This was our second night with no sleep.

Finally at around five in the morning, five and a half hours after the epidural, I had dilated to ten centimeters and was ready to push. The nurse called Dr. W and then instructed me as to when to push. It actually felt good at first. Dorothy, the nurse, was very encouraging and said I was doing a great job. I believed her. This encouragement gave me incentive and motivation to keep going. At one point, though, I remember feeling quite weird that people whom I didn't know, nurses and such, were walking in and out of my room. My bed faced the door, and I was spread-eagled facing the entrance. They could have given me some privacy or just introduced themselves when they walked in, like "Hi, vagina; how are you? I'm nurse so and so. Any heads emerging yet?"

After an hour or so of pushing and increasing the epidural, I started to feel pain again. They felt that the baby wasn't coming out fast enough as I approached two hours of pushing, so they inserted a vacuum suction, which was very painful. With a few more pushes and the help of the vacuum, the baby's head emerged with a hot, burning pain like nothing I can compare. With one big push, the rest of him gushed out, and I was relieved that it was finally over. I looked down and saw that it was a boy. Wow. My baby was out of me. I could finally meet this creature I had been dreaming about and wondering about for what seemed like so long.

They took him away quickly and suctioned him. I was glad that they warned me about this. I didn't think about him for a second; it was so sore and burning so much at the "baby exit." They cleaned him off, and he was okay. They wrapped him in a blanket and gave him to Rob. Rob brought him to me, and we looked into his beautiful eyes and said, "Hello, baby." We were in awe. He didn't cry; he just looked up at us with these big, dark, glossy eyes and almost smiled. He seemed to be taking it all in. Rob and I said to each other, "So do you still want to name him Skye Luka?" We both agreed. We had picked this name out and kept it secret from everyone. My labor was about thirty-one hours in total. Skye was born at 6:47 AM on August twelfth. He weighed seven pounds, six ounces and was twenty-one inches long.

After that, there was a harsh nurse was on shift. This woman was rough and abrupt. I kindly asked her to be careful with Skye because I felt she was not being gentle in handling him. Her response to me was a glaring stare as she said, "I've been doing this for a long time." When I wanted just a few moments to breastfeed Skye, she did not ask kindly if she could help me but snapped that there was a lot more to it than just putting him on. She tried to help me in an aggressive manner by trying to latch him on and then later said I refused to let her help me. She was also very focused on getting me showered and out of that room, and she was incredibly impolite about it. I felt humiliated and degraded when she had me walk over to the shower, a shower I didn't want to take until I got to my room, blood pouring down my legs and onto the floor. After my shower, as she forced a pad onto me in a fast and harsh manner, I had to say to her, "Don't! Please be gentle. It hurts."

When we got to the recovery room, she tried to take Skye away for more tests, and she all but grabbed him out of my arms. I wanted to hold him and preferred to wait for any further tests until after we'd had a chance to just be together. If the tests needed to be done immediately, I would have preferred for them to be done with him in my arms; however, I did not even have a chance to express my desires. The nurse raised her voice and told me they had to do the tests.

I felt like a little child in that wheelchair, humiliated and vulnerable. I had just had the most challenging and ecstatic experience of my life, and I was exhausted. I wanted to just revel in the moment with this new life. I said to her, "Please speak kindly to me." She peered down at me with anger on her face and said, "I'm a very kind person. You're very demanding, and you need to understand that we have rules and schedules to follow here." I said to her again, "All I'm asking is for you to speak kindly to me." She left in a huff without saying another word, and I burst into tears. I sobbed while I breastfed Skye for the first time, tears streaming onto his face.

I felt so alone. Rob saw it all and thought she was terrible, but he didn't say anything. I guess he felt he couldn't, or perhaps he was just shocked. I hoped Skye didn't sense the tension I was feeling. For over five weeks afterward, I had problems with breastfeeding. Skye would scream every time he was on the breast. I feel that this first negative experience may be connected with the problems I have experienced with breastfeeding. According to Dr. Jack Newman, a breastfeeding expert, it is very important to have your child on the breast within the first hour after birth. I also believe the epidural may have something to do with this as well.

During my labor I had no regrets about getting that epidural. But now that I look back, I wish I had had a doula or someone with experience there with me in the hospital. I wish someone could have fooled me into thinking that I would get drugs but then not actually have that happen. I wish I could have held out just a little longer because I was so close. I was starting to feel like the contractions were becoming pushing contractions. Over and over I replayed the events of my birthing experience. If I had chosen to birth naturally, I wouldn't have had such a terrible nurse when the shifts changed at seven AM. Skye might not have been so lethargic for twenty-four hours after his birth. He might have opened his mouth wider and latched on to the breast better had he not been drowsy. I might not have had such a tough time with extremely painful nursing.

I didn't realize any of this at the time, but by looking back, I now see what I didn't know then. I didn't know that an epidural would affect a baby quite that much, nor that it could interfere with breastfeeding. There was no mention of any possible side effects from the epidural for the baby or myself before it was administered. I am thankful that my baby was happy and healthy, but I have grieved over many losses and lost expectations. When I look back on my birth experience, I have cried many times and grieved over the one part of it that was most horrible: the way that nurse treated me at such an emotional and vulnerable time.

We got a private room in the hospital so Rob could stay overnight as well. The three of us snuggled on the tiny single bed. Rob and I slept sideways so we could have room. We didn't mind one bit. Sleep didn't happen for very long anyway. We loved having our son close and just enjoyed staring at him in awe. He looked so cute. His skin was dark and he was so beautiful. His eyes were captivating. I couldn't imagine Rob not being there. I needed his help with everything. Rob and Skye bonded right from the beginning. They now have a very close relationship built on a foundation that started from the moment Skye was born.

It was kind of nice in the hospital having meals prepared and all our laundry done for us. Diapers and lotion were provided for the baby. The annoying part was the invasion by the nurses: the tests and poking and prodding when I just wanted them to leave Skye and us alone. It all seemed unnecessary. Skye would be sleeping, and they'd stick a cold thermometer in his little armpit then say his temperature was too low and take him to the nursery to put him under the warmer. Then a different nurse would come along and say he was too warm.

We ended up spending four days in the hospital with help from the lactation consultant to get breastfeeding going. She was amazing. She treated me with dignity and respect. She was gentle, kind, and a refreshing welcome every day.

I still wished we had been at home for the whole event, as the transition from hospital to home was awful. I'm glad the lactation consultant warned us about this. The night we came home, Skye screamed until five thirty in the morning. He cried inconsolably for hours sometimes, and this went on for about three or four months.

I'm amazed at all a woman can go through mentally and physically. I thought I had done it all. I thought I was tough and adventurous, but labor showed me who I really was. Although I have struggled with guilt about taking medication, I felt I needed it to get through the intensity. I still dream of having a natural, unassisted home birth, and should we decide to have another child, I hope my dream will come true.

STACY SMITH'S BIRTH STORY

WHEN I FOUND out I was pregnant, I began planning and preparing for a natural childbirth—a birth without pain medication and with as little medical intervention as possible. I went through three health care providers before I found one I really trusted, and I read everything I could find on the topic, ending up with quite a collection of books on pregnancy and childbirth. I read every birth story I could get my hands on and spent a lot of time planning for, visualizing, and talking about what I hoped would be my perfect birth experience. Having been induced with my first daughter, I really wanted the experience of going into labor and birthing with as few interventions as possible. At my doctor's appointment right before my due date, my doctor said he wanted to talk about inducing labor with us after my due date had passed—and they were figuring my due date for the next Saturday. My husband and I talked and talked about it and decided that if we hadn't had a baby by the next Tuesday appointment, we would schedule the induction.

But I was still upset by the possibility of induction. It really wasn't what I wanted or what I planned on. I was praying daily that my body would know what to do, that the labor could start without interference and progress naturally. Not having experienced a unmedicated labor before, I was really struggling to have faith that I was capable of birthing my baby without medical assistance. The pregnancy hormones were in full force, and with just a few days to my due date, my emotions were definitely ruling my intellect. Logically, I knew I wouldn't be pregnant forever, but my due date came and found me sobbing that I didn't want to be pregnant anymore.

Saturday night I fell into bed exhausted. I slept okay that night (as okay as anyone does who is nine months pregnant!). I do remember waking up several times feeling kind of nauseous and crampy but figured it was probably dinner that wasn't agreeing with me. My twenty-month-old daughter, Abby, woke up really early Sunday morning, and we did all the stalling we could, but it was no use: we had to start the day. I wasn't feeling very well. My body was overtired and worn out, and I was physically incapable of doing much besides sitting on the living room couch.

It was a beautiful day outside. Our days were typical summer scorchers, but the morning was still cool, and the sky outside our window was sparkling blue with just a few clouds. After reading the same sentence four times without comprehending any of it, I laid my head back on the couch and started dozing a little bit. I noticed a contraction, but it felt like all the others had for the past few weeks: my belly started tightening involuntarily, and it gradually built up to a peak and then subsided. It wasn't painful or particularly intense, and I chalked it up to a Braxton Hicks contraction. I dozed off and then felt another contraction not too much later. I remember asking my husband Tom what time it was: nine-sixteen. I still wasn't too excited; I had had fairly regular contractions before and nothing ever came of it. I lay on the couch and waited for awhile but didn't feel any more contractions, so I decided it was probably time to start getting things ready for church.

Since Abby gave us all such an early wake-up call, I knew that she was going to be an exhausted and miserable toddler, so I brought her upstairs and rocked her for a little while, hoping that she would take an early nap and then be okay all through church. It didn't take long for her to fall asleep. We rocked and I sang some songs quietly. I remember feeling particularly close to her and very grateful for quiet moments together. She was laying her head against my chest with her hair falling across her closed eyes, and I started to feel pretty emotional. I had been aware for a few days that our time together as just the three of us was ending and that however wonderful it was going to be to have another person in our family and no matter how much our new daughter would be loved and cherished, things were never going to be the same. I realized that as our family dynamic shifted and Abby got older, there would be fewer and fewer quiet moments like this. When I moved her into her own bed for her nap, I knelt by her bed for a little while and rubbed her back, then leaned over and kissed her, loving the sight of my sweet daughter sleeping peacefully.

I woke up my tired husband, and we got in the shower together. I started feeling a few more contractions, still irregular and painless and most lasting less than thirty seconds. I told Tom what was happening, and he suggested staying home from church and seeing if we "could get things moving." I knew that if I stayed home expecting labor to start and then nothing happened, I would be terribly disappointed, and I had committed to playing the piano that day. As I was getting ready, I felt a few more light contractions, but didn't even bother timing them because I knew that when it was serious enough for me to start timing them I would know. After all, contractions are supposed to hurt, right? (Hah!)

I entered our church building and was immediately the focus of several well-intentioned but stupid comments like: "So, no baby yet?" I was tempted to respond, "Well, I really like being nine months pregnant, so I talked to the baby and convinced her to stay in a little longer." Because it was church, I bit back my sarcasm, smiled at them, rolled my eyes inwardly, and walked away. I listened through the children's service with my mind only half on what was being said. I had noticed that I was having quite a few contractions and started watching the clock. I raised my eyebrows a little bit when I realized that they were coming five minutes apart, almost exactly corresponding with the number on the clock: at eleven fifteen, at eleven twenty, at eleven twenty-five, and they kept coming regularly. Some lasted as long as forty-five seconds or so, but some were a little shorter, none of them hurt, and none of them were more than just a tightening sensation. When it was time for singing, I was having a hard time concentrating, mostly because I was watching the clock and anticipating the next contraction coming, interested to see if they would keep coming regularly. They were becoming a little more intense, and if I was playing a song during a contraction, I would inevitably miss a few more notes, and I wondered if anyone noticed that their piano player was falling apart!

I noticed that the contractions stopped when it came time for the one that was supposed to happen at eleven forty-five, and I didn't have one for about fifteen minutes after that. I was disappointed but thought that the contractions might start again later that day or the next. We had a short break, and I left my piano bench to stretch my legs and get a drink of water. I was standing by the water fountain when I felt my first hard contraction. It was an interesting feeling; I knew without a doubt this was a real contraction. This was more like a sharp, aching hurt in my pelvis, and although it didn't last very long, I definitely couldn't keep walking or do anything else during the contraction besides just stand there and breathe through it. I went back into the service but couldn't focus on anything that was being said and didn't have a prayer of finding a comfortable position on a piano bench! Before it was even time to play again, I knew I needed to go home. I was incredibly grateful at this point that I had decided to drive the short distance to church.

The contractions were powerful and came steadily all the way home. I could barely move or do anything else during the contractions and was completely annoyed that I had to get out of the van to open the gate. I knew at this point that I was either in labor or a very good imitation of it. I slowly walked in the house and was met by Abby running through the house at breakneck speed, with a huge grin on her face when she saw me. I yelled out to Tom that I was having some pretty serious contractions and that I thought that I was probably in labor. His eyes lit up and he began running around the house, finishing last-minute preparations.

The first thing I thought of was calling my parents. Their church started at one o'clock, and if I wanted to have someone to watch Abby when we needed to go to the hospital, I knew we needed to alert them. I was in the bedroom while Tom was on the phone with my mom. Another contraction hit, and I was kneeling on the floor, holding on to the bed. I could hear Tom tell my mom to take the cell phone to church, but after the contraction subsided, I said that someone needed to come now. I could tell that my contractions were building rapidly and figured that it would be time to leave for the hospital by the time a half hour passed and my mom arrived. Tom was asking me questions, but his voice and everything else going on around me faded into the background. All I could feel was this giant force within my body completely overtaking me, and I told him, rather sharply, not to talk to me until the contraction was over.

I tried going to the rocking chair in our front room. Kneeling on the floor and draping myself over the ottoman or the back of the rocking chair had been a huge help alleviating the back pain that I had experienced during my last trimester. Abby saw what I was doing and thought it was all a game—"Mom's spinning on the rocking chair!"—and tried to help me spin around. I yelled for Tom to come and get her. Luckily, when he called, she went running back down the hall.

When another contraction started, I had to moan through it; the sound just started coming out, almost involuntarily. Being in the rocking chair wasn't working, and I was frustrated because I couldn't seem to get control of the pain that I was feeling. When I had pictured being in labor, I had envisioned being in perfect control, meditative and quiet. Instead, I was pacing through the house like a noisy, frustrated animal, and one of the things that I thought would help the most didn't do a thing! The pains were coming faster than my ability to cope with them and I mentally searched for more options. The bathtub was the next thing that came to mind. I had pictured spending a lot of time in the hot water in labor, so I decided to give it a shot.

I told Tom I wanted him to fill the bath, and he hesitated, giving me an "I don't know about this" look, but thought better of it, and turned the water on. I got undressed, left my clothes all over the floor, and caught a glimpse of myself in the mirror, glad that I had done my hair and put on makeup that morning: I would look nice when I had this baby! (It's amazing the random, jumbled thoughts that came through my head between contractions!)

I got in the water and waited for the relief that everyone tells me they feel when they get in the water during labor. Nothing. I couldn't get comfortable for the life of me, and it seemed like every time I tried to shift positions, another contraction would start, leaving me powerless. Abby came in and, seeing me in the tub, started beaming. "Mama naked!" she said with glee. Then it was "Belly? Baby?" in her sweet voice, while touching my belly gently. Tears filled my eyes. I wondered briefly if she somehow knew what was about to happen, and I knew that my baby Abby wasn't going to be my baby much longer. I kissed her cheek gently and told her that Mama was going to have a baby today, and that I loved her so much, no matter what happened. Then I yelled for my husband to take her downstairs and put on a video for her or something. I couldn't handle such a distraction.

I was starting to get so irritated that I couldn't control my reaction to the contractions. During another break, I started to focus on some of the things I had read in Pam England's *Birthing from Within* about coping with pain. I had thought previously that unfocused awareness was something that would work well, and I had practiced it a lot, but when I tried to shut out what was going on and listen and observe as she advised, I couldn't do it. I was watching the shower curtain, trying to find a focus point, and couldn't get on top of the pain. I was still moaning, trying to keep it low pitched, but the moans were growing steadily higher and more intense. I felt something pop, saw some mucus floating in the tub, and then I felt my water release. A few seconds later I noticed that the water in the tub was turning slightly green and started to panic a little bit, knowing that there was meconium in the amniotic fluid.

Tom had just come back upstairs, and I breathlessly directed him where to find the number for the doctor on call for the weekend because I wanted to know what to do about the meconium. I heard him talking with the answering service and started getting really annoyed. Didn't they know that I was in labor? I wanted them to get the doctor now! I knew then that we needed to get to the hospital as soon as we could. In the next brief pause in between contractions, I told Tom we needed to leave for the hospital as soon as we could and he needed to go get someone from church to watch Abby.

Tom returned a lot quicker than I thought he would, and I was grateful. I really didn't want to be left alone anymore. I was starting to panic. I was so afraid that I was going to get to the hospital and have hours and hours of labor left to go. I wasn't coping well at all; I was overwhelmed by the sheer magnitude of the pain. I wondered why in the world I had thought natural childbirth was such a good idea. I wasn't enjoying this at all. I wasn't meditating or anticipating the birth like I had thought I would. I didn't feel beautiful or powerful. I was just in pain, and I wanted it to stop.

Tom brought Laura, a friend of ours from the neighborhood, and I was really grateful to hear her voice. The phone rang, and it was the doctor on call, and I could vaguely hear a conversation going on around me, but couldn't understand what was being said in the midst of another contraction. Tom tried to ask me how far apart the contractions were, and I yelled that they were right on top of each other. He then asked me if I could be a little more specific and in desperation, I just shouted that I'm sure they were less than two minutes apart.

Tom then came in and told me that I needed to get out of the tub. I couldn't imagine moving, but I knew that he was right. He helped me stand up, and was drying me off. He helped me into my pants and put a T-shirt over my head. Laura poked her head in when we told her I was decent (quite a time to be concerned about modesty!) and asked me what she could do. I wanted a drink of water, and she brought me one. Another contraction hit, and I dropped to my hands and knees on the bathroom floor, moaning. I felt like I was going to be ripped apart by this force. The pain was unlike anything I had ever felt or ever imagined. It was centered deep inside my pelvis and radiated everywhere.

I cried out that I couldn't do it anymore, that I didn't want to do it. Laura was rubbing my back and shoulders and told me that I could do it, and that I was doing it. She then said that she thought I was in transition, and I would have laughed at the idea if I physically could have. There was no way I was in transition. I had not been in labor long enough! I was seriously worried about how much longer I could handle the pain. At that point I was ready to throw all plans for natural birth out the window. An epidural sounded like heaven to me, although the moaning with the next contraction came from the knowledge that I still had to get to the hospital (about a half hour away) and get admitted before they could do anything.

I decided it was time to start moving toward the van, and the two of them helped me up slowly, and we started walking to car. I was literally hanging on Tom's neck during the next contraction and was pleasantly surprised to find that it relieved some of the intensity. What a time to find a position that worked!

I decided to kneel on the front seat of our van and drape my arms around the back of the seat. Concerned for my safety, Tom put the seatbelt around the back of me, which I thought was pretty silly. I rode for a few minutes that way, but I was so hot. I asked if the air conditioning could be turned on any higher, but it was already going at full blast. I couldn't handle how hot I was feeling, so I had to turn around. Tom was speeding through our residential neighborhood at about fifty miles per hour, honking his horn as he went.

I was trying so hard to get comfortable in my seat and get focused. Tom gave me the hand that he wasn't driving with, and I started squeezing that for all I was worth. I was literally screaming at this point. There was nothing else I could do. We had just made a turn onto a major street, when I felt the baby's head drop into my birth canal. "The baby's coming!" I screamed. I don't know how I knew it, it sounded bizarre and ridiculous, but instinctively I knew that she was really close.

Tom told me, very calmly, "No, we are going to the hospital. We'll be there in about twenty minutes." With the next contraction, my body started to push. At first, I didn't recognize the sensation. It felt like I was about to have a huge bowel movement, and I thought, briefly, how embarrassed I would be if that happened. But the feeling got stronger and stronger, and with the next contraction, I knew that my body was pushing this baby out and there wasn't anything I could do to stop it. Cooperating with it and pushing was the only thing I could do. Whoever described it as the "urge" to push really didn't do that feeling justice! It's more like an overwhelming and uncontrollable force, a tidal wave. Fighting against it was impossible.

I screamed again: "I'm pushing; my body is pushing!" and Tom responded back, "I don't know what to do!" I told him to stop the van, and he kept going. I hit him on the arm and screamed again that I was pushing. Again he said that he didn't know what to do, and I screamed at him to "Pull over and dial 911!"

We had just pulled onto the highway and pulled off to the shoulder of the road. He told me I had to let go of his hand so that he could dial, and I was barely aware of letting go. Once again I had that odd feeling of having a conversation go on around me without being able to understand what was said. The force that was going through me was absolutely amazing. I was pushing with every contraction, and the relief from the intensity of the contractions was coupled with the primal, instinctive effort that was going to bring my baby into the world.

Before I knew it, Tom had come around to my side of the van and was trying to persuade me to take my pants off. I'm still not sure how I managed that feat, sitting in the front seat of a minivan while having contractions. He looked down between my legs and announced to the 911 dispatcher that he could see the head. I think that was when it really hit me: we were going to have the baby right there on the freeway. I started to feel burning, stinging, and in the back of my mind remembered the "ring of fire" and realized that she was crowning. There was no way I could think myself through this. My body was completely in control. My whole mind, body, and soul were consumed with the power and force of each contraction. It was amazingly primal and powerful.

Tom put his hand on my perineum on the instructions of the dispatcher, but I felt my body push against his hand, like it was rebelling against his restriction, and all of a sudden, her head was out. Tom reached down to get a towel to wipe her face and mouth when a final huge contraction came rippling through my body like a wave and I heard him say, "She's out, she's out, she's all the way out!" I couldn't believe it—my baby had been born. I felt a huge rush of adrenaline, knowing that labor was over and reached for my baby, begging to hold her.

Tom put my little girl on my chest and it was one of the most powerful, emotional moments of my life. I looked at this little body and was completely amazed that she had been inside me only a few seconds before. She wasn't crying, but was a perfect shade of pink, so I knew that she was breathing. She was wrapped up in our big purple beach towel and was wet, with a little smear of blood on her eyebrow. She was still in my arms, looking up at me with these wide, intense, darker-than-dark eyes, like she was as amazed as I was at what had just happened to her.

I was filled with this overpowering love for her. There is nothing in the world that could compare to that moment. I studied every inch of her that I could see: her tiny hands, her thick, dark hair, and the still pulsing umbilical cord, which was surprisingly long and thin. Here was this tiny little person who had just come from inside me. She seemed so much smaller than I remember babies being, and so incredibly beautiful. Tom was still on the phone with the dispatcher, and I watched him tie off the umbilical cord with his shoelace. It seemed like the minute he cinched it tight, we heard the sirens of the ambulance, and we both breathed a sigh of relief.

Before I knew what had happened, there were four paramedics looking in on us, three men and a woman who looked at me, smiled, and said, "Hi, mom, we're going to take care of you." I could have hugged her. It was so nice knowing that someone else was in control. They quickly cut the baby's cord, and I saw some of the blood spurt out onto my arm. I felt a small pang as they took her from me, as were being separated for the first time in nine months. Two of the paramedics loaded me carefully onto a stretcher, and for the first time, I became aware that there were cars whizzing by on the freeway, and I was naked from the waist down. How bizarre that I had just participated in such a life-changing event and yet life was going on as normal for all these people around me!

They loaded us both into the ambulance, and I was lying on the stretcher in a daze, trying to process everything that had happened in the last few minutes. They started an intravenous line and put an oxygen mask on me, neither of which I wanted, but didn't have the energy to fight. I realized I was feeling contractions again and I was so angry: I had forgotten that I still had a placenta to deliver. They gave me the baby to try and nurse, but lying on a stretcher in the back of an ambulance was not the ideal place to begin our nursing relationship. The baby nuzzled with me a little bit, but they wanted her to stay so covered up and have an oxygen mask nearby, so it just wasn't working. They decided to leave the placenta until we got to the hospital because the contractions weren't doing anything and they wanted the obstetrician to deal with it.

When we got to the hospital, they put the baby on my chest all wrapped up, and we were wheeled through the hospital on the stretcher. I got a kick out of all the curious looks and stares we got as we were wheeled through the emergency room, the halls, and then up the elevator. We got up to the labor and delivery floor, and two nurses immediately jumped up when they saw us, following all of us into a labor and delivery room.

Everyone seemed concerned that I hadn't delivered the placenta yet, and I was getting more and more frustrated because it seemed so unfair to do all this work to get the baby out and then have to have more contractions. At one point, I had a nurse applying pressure to my uterus and one trying to pull on the umbilical cord, but it still wouldn't come. They decided to call the obstetrician on call, and he went straight to work. I wanted to deliver the placenta so badly at this point. I just wanted the contractions to stop! During the next few contractions, I was pushing with everything I had, and finally, finally, almost an hour after the baby was born, the placenta was delivered.

Then it was time for the stitching. This was, quite literally, more painful than the contractions leading up to the birth. I didn't know it at the time, but I had a second-degree tear toward my rectum, and then had torn upward straight through my urethra, and through my clitoris. The next half hour or so, while the doctor was stitching me up, was absolutely excruciating. I was aware of every stitch, even with pain medication, and it felt like they were tearing me apart at the most sensitive places possible. I learned later that the paramedics said that I looked like I had a gunshot wound, and the doctor said it looked like I had sat on a hand grenade. I'm glad that they didn't tell me that until after I had been stitched up!

Periodically a nurse came in with updates on the baby. We found out she weighed six pounds, fourteen ounces and that she was nineteen and a half inches long. They had to take her to the NICU (neonatal intensive care unit) because her core temperature was low, but I would get to see her as soon as I could. The doctor on call finally made it in soon afterward and reassured me that he would do everything he could to get me back together with the baby. That was the only thing that made any sense after all the pain I had gone through. I wanted to hold her, see her, touch her, and nurse her. Finally, the nurses told me that I could be wheeled to the NICU, and they took me to see my daughter.

The first thing I saw when I was rolled in the door was my husband in a rocking chair, holding our little daughter and talking to her softly. Tears came to my eyes, and I reached for her. She was so beautiful.

We became minor celebrities for the whole time we were in the hospital. Every nurse, assistant, lab person, or anyone who came into the room seemed to know exactly who we were and wanted to hear details of the story. I laughed when we were wheeled into the room and saw that a message had been written on the white board: "Congratulations, Mom and Dad, on the speedy delivery. Hope your daughter doesn't spend her whole life living in the fast lane!"

⟡

REIKO JODI HALPERIN'S BIRTH STORY

IF I HAD only known then what I know now, I would not have used drugs. My first two birthing experiences were drug induced, but my third was very empowering because I was enlightened with knowledge. Most of my friends who delivered without medication did so because their labor came on rapidly. I don't believe these same friends would choose to repeat their scenarios. I desired to have a choice in matters pertaining to my body. So when I became pregnant for the third time, I elected to do a bit of research.

Orange County, where I live, is not the mecca for holistic ideas. It is a conservative county with many moms driving jumbo SUVs, soccer moms, and numerous corporate entities on every street corner. What this means for the expectant mother is that there are numerous scheduled deliveries via caesarean and many medicated births. Such is this norm that my male obstetrician gave me a funny chuckle when I mentioned that I was researching ways to deliver the baby without medication. He said, "I wish the epidural was available when my wife delivered our babies years ago."

My first eye-opening venture came through reading the book *Ina May's Guide to Childbirth*. Thank goodness I came across this well-written book at my local library. It challenged many ideas that I had taken for granted: that doctors knew what was best for their patients and that pain should be eradicated. Ina May's book suggests that the way the U.S. media presents labor pains is brainwashing the general public. On a worldwide scope, it is believed that labor pain is a normal and expected part of childbirth and that women can cope with the contractions. But in the United States, the media bombards us with screaming women in labor, their legs in stirrups, while their husbands have that panicked deer in the headlights look. It is no wonder that first-time mothers are apprehensive about the whole birthing experience. This expectation of pain causes severe anxiety that often itself causes pain because anxiety actually causes the body and the mind to tighten up.

Another idea that is perpetuated is that a laboring mother should not be allowed to eat or drink during labor. But how is the laboring mother going to have the energy to go through the contractions and push? Heck, it just makes sense that women should be gearing their bodies for labor by consuming light snacks and liquids, as any athlete would do during a marathon. Again, Ina May's book introduced concepts that made me rethink my doctor's practice. My first labor lasted seventeen hours, and I was not allowed to have a lollipop or even chew gum. The nurse said, "Only ice chips." Instead of concentrating on my labor, I became fixated on what I would drink and eat after the baby was born. When my sister-in-law arrived to visit our baby, she showed up with four bottles of sparkling fruit cider. I was just as relieved to quench my thirst as I was that my labor was completed.

Another idea in Ina May's book is that during labor the mother should keep moving to help labor along, and the birthing class we attended mentioned that too. But if the mother is given a labor-inducing medicine and hooked up to an intravenous line, she must remain in bed and be monitored. This dogmatic rule wasn't mentioned in our birthing class. Furthermore, with all the epidural in my body, labor slowed down and I was in danger of having a caesarean. Luckily the caesarean was not needed when I finally dilated seventeen hours later. Because I felt numb from the waist down, I was not pushing effectively with the contractions, which caused me to push for two hours and end up with an episiotomy and stitches. The doctor gave me a mirror to help me push the head out, but I was so extremely frustrated, thirsty, and tired that the mirror was more of a hindrance than an aid.

Happily, everything was okay considering the arduous labor and delivery. My baby was very healthy and weighed eight pounds, six ounces. Being a first-time mother, I did not know what to expect after the birth. The lingering side effects were very frightening. My upper body shook for an hour, and the stitches from the episiotomy made me very upset. Furthermore, I could not stand up for several hours. No one warned me that I would shake for two hours and that I wouldn't be able to hold my daughter. The cause may have been the drugs in my system; I had both pitocin and the epidural. Although my baby seemed content and nursed right away, I wondered if the drugs were causing her to be extremely lethargic. The side effects of the drugs were transmitted into her system through my breast milk. My obstetrician could not give me a definitive answer about the cause of my side effects.

The second time we were expecting, I talked to a mother who had taken a hypnosis class, and I was intrigued. But life took over, and we just repeated the same old birthing class offered by the hospital. We didn't learn anything new, and it just seemed a big waste of time. I was scared to go through labor again. I knew what the drugs did to my system last time, and I did not think I could "breathe through the contractions." The only consolation I had was that second deliveries are much faster, or so other mothers told me.

The second delivery was uneventful except for some unsolicited advice a stranger gave me during my admission into the emergency room. We got admitted at one AM, and this man took one look at me and said one word: "Epidural." Did I look that desperate and pained? Well, I must have been easily influenced, because as soon as I got into the labor and delivery room, the nurse gave me the epidural. My husband and I took a two-hour nap and woke up refreshed. Then it was time to push, and our second daughter was born within thirty minutes. How easy was that? But that was only the beginning of the ordeal.

Unknown to us she was born with a diaphragmatic hernia. My obstetrician thought that the trauma of the pushing caused her small intestines to push into her upper diaphragm, or else that it was probably a late-term development that had not been detected. Again, I didn't get to hold my baby because I was shaking so hard from the drugs, and then she was immediately taken away to the children's hospital for X-rays and monitoring. I didn't get to fully bond with her until nine days later. She came out of surgery fine, but that first night after her birth was a nightmare. Not only was I alone in my bed without my newborn baby, but my arm swelled so badly that I could not sleep. I have never felt so helpless in my entire lifetime. I vowed to never be at the mercy of medication again.

Two years later when we were expecting our third baby, I kept my promise and pursued my research into a safer birthing. My research led me to investigate a hypnosis tape program led by Kerry T., and it was well worth the investment in time and energy. I was committed to trying the program if only I could get over my skepticism. I am afraid of pain, and just the thought of pain made me stressful. But I put my faith in myself and got my act together. My husband and I listened to the tapes and practiced diligently from my seventh month to the night of my labor. It was not easy to be different from the other expecting parents, but we had a detailed birth plan that I devised. The labor nurse respected our wish to use the hypnosis tapes and the birthing ball. I was expecting a different birthing, but I had no idea how fast everything would flow.

Our journey began at twelve thirty AM when my water broke. We checked into the hospital at one AM, and I started to visualize the perfect birth. I started to incorporate the birthing program as soon as I was in the labor and delivery room. I bounced around on my big silver birthing ball and focused as much as I could. I stopped dilating for two hours, and this was when I started to feel disappointment creeping into my thoughts. Maybe my body did require the pitocin as in the two previous births. But I was determined to give it one hundred percent total gumption. I bounced on the birthing ball for thirty continuous minutes. I started to feel more uncomfortable and had the labor nurse check me. Hurray! I was starting to make progress and dilated to eight centimeters.

Then everything went just a little too fast. I needed to go to the bathroom right away. The nurse requested that I only urinate. Luckily, my husband assisted me into the bathroom because I started to panic. I needed to push right there on the toilet. The nurse called the front desk right away for a doctor. I barely made it onto the bed when the urge came again. I said, "The baby is coming now!" During the other two birthings, my husband and the staff cheered, "Push!" However, this time they kept saying, "Don't push!" During the other two birthings I hollered, "Please get the baby out now!" But this birthing was different; I was in control.

This is when my husband knew the hypnosis was working. When I couldn't stop the wave of panic overcoming my mind, he gave me the cue that we had practiced. Just then he could see my whole body relaxing and a renewed sense of calmness overtook me. I also felt a renewed sense of determination that I could and would complete this delivery the natural way. The doctor barely had enough time to prep his equipment when my baby girl just slid out of my body. I don't even think I pushed or struggled to get her to move down the birth canal. It was surreal that it happened so fast. I did it! I delivered my third baby just the way I envisioned I would. My husband was so proud of our accomplishment that he shared our story with our closest friends and family and anyone else who would listen.

The best part, of course, was that because I had a natural birthing, I held my baby right away. I felt like I was able to bond with this baby immediately after the birth, rather than sometime later as with my first two babies. I felt a little tired, but I was able to drink, stand up, and be mobile. I felt extremely proud of myself, and my husband was elated that to be part of such an awesome experience. He felt like a participant in his daughter's delivery instead of a bystander in the room. The experience was such an emotional high that one hour afterward, I looked deeply into his hazel eyes and said, "Let's have another baby."

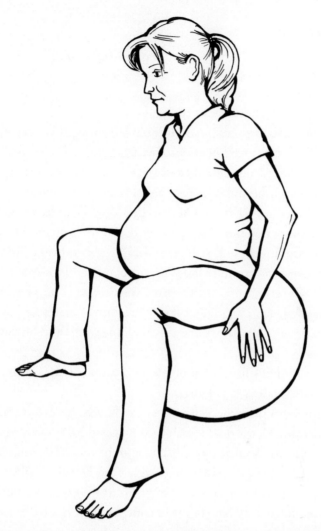

SITTING UPRIGHT is an optimal position throughout pregnancy, labor, and birth. Labors where the woman is vertical are aided by the force of gravity and by the power of contractions focusing on the cervix. Having the legs open expands the pelvis and gives the baby space to maneuver and engage. Using a birthing ball instead of a regular chair adds a new dimension because the ball is soft to the perineum and it allows the woman to gently rock and roll in place with the rhythm of the contraction. Sitting comfortably on the birthing ball helps the woman's back and pelvis stay loose while supporting the perineum. The flexible ball feels softer and more stable if it is somewhat deflated. Letting some air out of the ball also allows the woman to place her feet firmly on the floor. She can rest while sitting on the ball, gently rocking and rolling in place, and relax in between contractions, disconnecting her attention from her surroundings and reaching a point of contemplation. This "trance" is necessary; otherwise, rational thoughts will prevent the woman's body from truly relaxing and working without obstruction.

⚬

KAREN YATES'S BIRTH STORY

I FIRST LEARNED of hypnosis for childbirth from a girlfriend who had used it as her birthing method. She showed me a videotape of when she was dilated to seven centimeters and in hard labor. On the tape she was sitting in a cushy leather chair with headphones on, eyes closed, head slumped over on her shoulder. She looked asleep. Her husband, holding the video camera, scrolled over to the contraction monitor and we watched with awe as the line curved sharply upward, higher and higher, signifying a significant birthing surge that lasted over three minutes long. My husband and I looked at each other dumbfounded and enthusiastically said, "We want what she's having."

I grew up with a serious phobia of needles, doctors, and hospitals, so Curtis and I began praying for a quick and easy birthing from the moment we found out I was pregnant. Now, I had heard other people say that they, too, were afraid of needles, but since the age of seven every doctor's appointment involving a blood test, shot, or even physical examination usually resulted in my fainting and/or hyperventilating. This was beyond a fear for me; it was a serious medical dilemma. How would I be able to give birth consciously? How would I handle the blood? Would they be able to find the vein for an intravenous needle, and would I be strong enough to push out our beautiful baby?

Let me put my fainting episodes into context so you understand the seriousness of our dilemma. I have fainted in movies, at every job I've ever worked, during college, and even at the bank and the grocery store. I've had doctors research why this happens to me, and from what they've explained, my body faints as a defense mechanism to pain, fear, worry, or stress. I have gotten to a point where I can usually tell I am about to pass out, and no matter where I am, I will lay myself down on the ground. Even if I am in the middle of a shopping mall, I will lay myself down. (In high school twice I fainted from a standing position and it was not pretty.)

Complicating my body's physical response to fear was my mental inability to cope with knowing ahead of time that I was going to faint. It was a cyclical battle. I would anticipate a blood test and faint before the needle pricked my skin. I would think of childbirth and have nightmares that I was not going to perform well during our birthing. I would think of pushing a baby out of me and start to experience precursors to fainting. My anxiety over childbirth was causing my body to physically collapse into exactly what I hoped to avoid.

I had blood tests, internal exams, and pain ahead of me, and I wanted to be ready. Although I had many friends advise, "just get the epidural," I was actually more afraid of the IV and the epidural than I was of the pain of childbirth. I hoped hypnosis could take me to a place where I could let go of these fears, let go of the "what ifs," and simply dream about my beautiful baby.

We began a class with Hypnobabies that was positive and uplifting. We started to look forward to the day we could meet our baby rather than dread it. Every night we practiced our hypnotapes, learning how to enter into a deep, relaxed state of mind. These tapes taught me to embrace my pregnancy, to breathe deeply, and to go to a special, safe place in my thoughts. Later we began to practice self-anesthetizing, and I learned to send anesthesia to the core of my body by simply telling my body to administer it. After a few months I had taught myself to shut off all fear, anxiety, and worry and to turn on all blessing, hope, and gratefulness. It was a critical mind shift that would prove essential to my birthing experience.

About five months into my pregnancy, I was able to test my hypnosis training when I walked through a blood test with more courage than ever before. Although I had tears in my eyes, I did not faint for the first time in twenty years.

Hypnobabies taught me to meditate on the positive rather than the negative, and by the time our due date arrived, I was ready. I had never felt more prepared for what was before me. When my water broke at eleven AM on September seventeenth, I called Curtis, happy and encouraged. Together we dallied around the house throughout the day, waiting for my birthing surges to get close together. At two AM when we arrived at the hospital, I was dilated to three centimeters. Although we had hoped to avoid an intravenous line, they did start one because they didn't want to risk infection. I did not cry, and I did not faint. By twenty-four hours into my labor, I was dilated to five centimeters on no medication, walking around the hospital in what I would call mild discomfort. I took a nap that afternoon, in the middle of labor, again with no medication. Because things were progressing slowly, thirty hours into my labor the hospital staff decided to start me on a pitocin drip. For nearly six hours, I received pitocin in an attempt to "kick start" my body into more aggressive labor. But it was to no avail.

Sure, we were frustrated. For thirty-six hours we struggled to have our baby, trying every natural technique we could. We wanted an easy birthing. We wanted a quick, pain-free, smooth day. But God had something else in mind.

Finally our doctors advised a caesarean section. They believed that our child might be too large to pass through the birth canal. So we agreed, and at 11:47 PM, thirty-seven hours after my water had broken, our son Zach was born, weighing a whopping ten pounds eleven ounces!

Now, did hypnosis work? I would argue that yes, it absolutely worked. I made it through hours of labor without fainting. In fact, in the throes of labor I was laughing, calmly sipping on juice, strolling around dilated to five centimeters on no medication, taking a nap, brushing my hair. Me?! Me who hates hospitals, doctors, and IVs. Me who fainted during the movie *Braveheart* nearly a dozen times. Me who once collapsed after a shot of Benadryl. And then to courageously undergo a caesarean section without a thought! I owe my calm, rational, and positive birthing experience to hypnosis.

Birthing naturally with a doula

Claudia Villeneuve

For a long time I did not believe that we needed doulas, because we had midwives. But it is clear that if women are to have one-to-one support, they cannot rely on it coming from busy midwives in a high tech hospital [or busy home birth practice], and that though agreed goals for midwifery include continuity of care and sensitive awareness of every woman's needs, at present this cannot be guaranteed. —Sheila Kitzinger[1]

What is a doula?

Having an experienced person offer continuous emotional and physical support to a woman during labor and birth is one of the greatest rediscoveries of modern obstetrics. This experienced person is called a doula or a paramana-doula, which means woman serving woman. Doula is a Greek word loosely translated to mean "woman's servant" or "minister to the woman." It has come to refer to professional labor and/or postpartum support for the birthing family. The care provider, doctor or midwife, provides the clinical skills, freeing the doula to provide the emotional support that the woman needs.

Birth assisting or birth supporting is a tradition thousands of years old. Traditionally, when a woman went into labor, other women in her community were expected to come to her home and help. This social expectation had the added benefit of exposing childless women to the experience of birth. The idea of mothering the mother is not new; what is new is the statistical evidence of how effective this kind of support is.

From the book *Mothering the Mother: How a Doula Can Help You Have a Shorter, Easier, and Healthier Birth* by Klaus et al., if you really desire it and are determined to achieve it, having a doula results in:

- a fifty percent reduction in caesarean rates
- a twenty-five percent reduction in average length of labor
- a sixty percent reduction in requests for an epidural
- a forty percent reduction in the use of oxytocin (Pitocin) to induce labor
- A thirty percent reduction in analgesia use
- A forty percent reduction in forceps deliveries

It is an understatement to say that women need support, beyond medical support, during the powerful and sometimes overwhelming experience of birth. Dr. Michel Odent, a French obstetrician and midwife who for years has conducted research on the physiological needs of laboring women, agrees with other researchers such as John Kennel, Phyllis Klaus, and Marshall Klaus that women experience shorter and better labors when they receive focused emotional and physical support. Births with doulas resulted in shortened labors and little need for medical intervention including artificial oxytocin, epidural anesthesia, and caesarean sections.

It was the level of support that had the greatest influence on outcomes. Therefore, when women and their families search for natural birth options, having a doula should be at the top of the list.

What I found most helpful from my doula was the hands-on comfort measures provided when I needed them; for example, hugs, massage, applying heating pads to my back, holding my hand, etc., as well as the constant verbal reassurances that I was "strong and capable to birth vaginally" and telling me how great I was doing and helping me to breathe and stay calm and relaxed during contractions. We truly worked together as a team: me, baby, husband, doula, and midwife. My husband most definitely welcomed the presence of a doula. He valued her support as much as I did. This was an emotionally charged experience for him as well. I believe that if doulas had been available to me fifteen and eleven years ago, the outcome of those births would have been different—possibly vaginal rather than all Caesarean deliveries. —DENISE ISKIW, who chose a doula for her vaginal birth after three caesareans

A doula is trained and/or experienced in the emotional, psychological, and physiological processes of birth. The doula's role is to look out exclusively for the emotional well-being of the mother. A birth doula does not replace a doctor or midwife and will not do vaginal exams or check blood pressure.

Some doulas see themselves as the protector of the mother's memories of the birth, so they ensure that the mom receives the best emotional care. More than the physical trauma, the emotional trauma is what builds disappointing birth memories. The doula supports the mother with constant attention to her needs—food, drink, massage, comforting words, and trust in her capacity to birth.

Photographs are also in the realm of a doula's work. She can take the photos that the parents cannot take because they are immersed in the labor. A doula can sense which moments of the labor and birth should be captured.

Other doulas see themselves as cheerleaders. The experiences of labor and birth can be overwhelming, and having a person who trusts in your capacity to give birth and in the normalcy of birth can keep you motivated. Women like to be surrounded by women who trust them. It is a sixth sense of knowing what another woman needs that can make a doula very useful.

Doulas are not labor coaches. A coach would bench you if you didn't perform. A doula is trained to provide:

- explanations of medical procedures
- emotional support
- advice during pregnancy
- exercise and physical suggestions to make pregnancy more comfortable

- help with preparation of a birth plan
- massage and other nonpharmacological pain relief measures
- suggestions for positioning during labor and birth
- support to the partners so that they can love and encourage the laboring woman
- alternatives to unnecessary interventions

The doula delivers continuity of care from home to hospital, easing the transition into the hospital environment, being there through changing hospital shifts and alternating physician schedules, serving as advocate, and supporting the partner to give the parents-to-be the freedom to focus inward as they meet the challenges and rewards of their birthing experience. She may be trained in and use birth art, meditation, birth hypnosis, relaxation, massage for labor, aromatherapy, lactation, and other modalities.

A doula's training can come from a variety of sources, usually including local training programs run by childbirth professionals, hospitals, birthing centers, or colleges; or from experience as a volunteer doula in a hospital or other birth setting. Some doulas are aspiring or apprenticing midwives, childbirth educators, or birth professionals. Others are trained through a national organization such as Birthworks, Association of Labor Assistants and Childbirth Educators (ALACE), International Childbirth Education Association (ICEA), Lamaze, or Doulas of North America (DONA).

Depending on where you live, finding a doula may be a challenge. Contact your local pregnancy and birth resource center, if you have one. You can also contact the following resources in your area for names of doulas:

- La Leche League leader
- independent childbirth educator
- local midwife
- local hospital
- birth center
- women's resource center
- natural foods/vitamin store resource board
- national doula organizations (listed in the resources at the end of this chapter)

Many doulas will come to your home in early labor and assist you to labor at home with confidence and support. If you are birthing in a hospital or birth center, the doula will then accompany you and continue to support you there.

~·~

How can you have a natural birth with a doula?

How do you expect women to prepare for natural childbirth? I expect them to prepare for it their whole lives. Unfortunately, our Westernized society doesn't prepare women very well. Therefore, mature, strong, independent women do not believe they can achieve a natural childbirth. The best preparation might be for her to attend several births before her own. Obviously, this may not be practical for everyone. Another important step is to choose a birth place that will not interfere with labor unnecessarily and create the need for medical support. She needs a caregiver who inspires confidence in her and who treats the emotional side as well as the physical. A doula can offer that. —KAREN WIRTANEN, doula, instructor for Birthing from Within

HAVING A DOULA actively helping the mother or even just sitting quietly in the room during labor significantly reduces requests for pain medication. In some cases, the epidural request rate was reduced by as much as sixty percent. Since delaying or simply refusing an epidural can decrease the risk of a caesarean section, doulas can help mothers achieve vaginal birth after caesarean (VBAC) or avoid caesareans altogether.

It is very important that obstetrical interventions are avoided as much as possible since one intervention can lead to other interventions, known as the cascade of obstetrical interventions. Getting an epidural to let you sleep during labor leads to needing an intravenous line, a catheter, and a Pitocin drip. Once you have an epidural, you might not be allowed to get off the bed because of hospital policy requiring a nurse or two to stay with you in case you fall. Staying

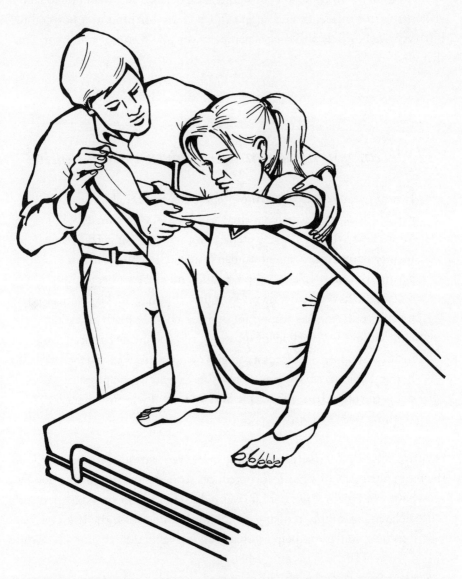

THE SQUATTING BAR on a hospital bed is a great tool for birth. When people choose a hospital or birth center, they should ask if squatting bars are available and whether or not they will be allowed to deliver while squatting. Midwives and enlightened physicians are comfortable catching babies while women squat. As well, the woman can see her baby being born. The bar is firm and fits and locks in the bed and can be adjusted for a woman's height by adding cushions to sit on.   Squatting can open up the pelvis 30 percent, which can make a difference in avoiding episiotomy, forceps, vacuum, and caesarean section. Invasive interventions like these add pain and health risks to the recovery period after the birth.

in bed means that now the uterus, the pelvis, and the baby are not in an optimal vertical position for efficient laboring and birth. This may lead to a long pushing stage, which might lead to forceps, vacuum cup, or even caesarean delivery.

Mothers who are determined to have a natural birth need a doula for additional support and would certainly enjoy the pampering they offer. Here's a formula for a safe and natural birth:

> Determined mom
> + Doula
> + Enlightened physician or midwife
> ———————————————
> A safe, natural birth

All the elements in this equation work together to create the proper environment for a birth that is safe and natural.

An enlightened physician is one who understands that birth is a normal process and that obstetrical interventions should be reserved for emergencies. You can expect little or no help from a physician who is not enlightened and is not working on your side to fully support your quest for a drug-free birth. In such a situation, your opportunity to have a natural birth may be compromised, even if you have a doula. The physician, following standard protocols of practice, will suggest a list of interventions to speed up the labor and birth. In this case a lay person without medical training (and in the middle of contractions) is not able to provide informed consent.

A doula can explain the procedures that the physician is suggesting, but the doula cannot tell the physician or the mother what to do. In fact, the doula cannot intervene in the relationship between the physician and the mother the way a husband might. The husband can discuss with the physician the need for these interventions and request, with the mother's approval, that they are not undertaken, but a doula cannot. She can tell you what would help you have a natural birth, but she cannot make the decision for you. A doula is an advocate for the mother to the extent that she will support a mother's decision in front of the medical staff. However, it is ultimately the mother who faces the final decision to say "yes, please" or "no, thanks."

Even though you may have an enlightened physician or a midwife, you still need continuous support, beginning when the first signs of labor appear.

Continuous support cannot be supplied by a physician in a busy hospital or by a midwife with a busy practice. They may want to provide it, but their advanced training and expertise is better suited to actually delivering babies, not offering support during what could be a long labor. Such support can be provided by a suitably trained and/or experienced doula. During the process of pushing out the baby, the physician and the midwife shift their attention to the baby, not the mom. At this critical point, the doula stays with the mother.

Doulas don't catch babies; they catch moms. They support mothers in any way that is needed. In the process they catch dads too. Many times the dad is the one person truly lost in the birthing experience. He doesn't have birthing hormones running through his veins to keep him focused, and no one offers him so much as an aspirin. Doulas help by involving dads in the process.

To have a natural birth with a doula, first become clear about what kind of birth you desire, choosing a caregiver and a place of birth. If you have those decisions in place, a doula can support you on your journey. The following scenario presents the basic picture of how a doula supports a mother in a hospital who is determined to have a natural birth:

> The mother hires a doula because she wants a natural birth; she wants control of her birthing experience. The mother chooses a doctor that her sister recommended because he was supportive of her successful vaginal birth after caesarean.
>
> When labor begins, the doula and the mother labor calmly at home for the first few hours. They use a hot shower, a bath, and counterpressure massage to cope with the contractions. The contractions get closer together until they are four minutes apart for over an hour. The mother wants to stay at home a little bit longer because she wants to avoid being in the hospital longer than necessary. The mother gets on hands and knees and begins rocking from side to side while the doula offers her a drink of juice. When the mother decides to go to the hospital, the father drives the car while the doula rides in the back seat with the mom, talking softly to her during the contractions.
>
> After being admitted to the hospital, the mother tells the nurse that she is prepared to accept a minimum amount of electronic

fetal monitoring while standing up. The nurse offers to start an intravenous line, but the mother tells her that she will have drinks so that will not be unnecessary. When the physician suggests oxytocin to augment the labor that he says is slow, the mother asks for time to make a decision. When alone, she discusses it with her doula, who will probably say that she knows many natural ways of augmenting labor: standing up, walking briskly, using nipple stimulation, sitting on the toilet, squatting, etc. When the physician comes back, the mother tells him that she needs more time to try other methods and that as long as the baby's heartbeat is doing fine, she is prepared to be in labor as long as necessary.

If the nurse offers an epidural to help the mother relax and even sleep, the mother asks for time to think about it. When alone the mother discusses it with her doula, who will probably say that she knows many natural ways of lowering the pain and helping the mother relax: a warm shower, a warm bath, massage or hip squeeze and counterpressure, aromatherapy, birthing ball, visualization, etc. Again when the nurse returns, the mother tells her that she needs more time to try other methods and that as long as the baby's heartbeat is doing fine, she is prepared to be in labor as long as necessary.

Within an hour the mother feels like pushing, and she decides to give birth in the squat position, using the squatting bar of the hospital bed. Her doula is right next to her, offering words of encouragement and holding her up next to the squat bar. The baby is born into the physician's hands, and the mother gets to experience and feel everything. The baby is wide awake, and they put him into the mother's arms right away.

We see in this scenario that the doula has given the woman excellent support by explaining treatment options, continuous following the mother's birth plan, communicating trust in her body's capacity to give birth, and faith in the normalcy of birth. This is what a determined mom needs to get the job done naturally.

❦

Why do parents choose a doula?

THERE ARE MANY reasons why parents choose a doula to accompany them at the birth. The most common one is to have a natural and satisfying birth experience. The phenomenon of new consumerism among educated and well-informed parents claiming their right to determine the course of their birth experience is the result of years of hospital interventions and procedures that modernized birth but in the process dehumanized its participants.

> I was also afraid I might forget everything I learned in my class (which I did!).

Generally, birth assistants are used by people having their baby in the hospital, but desiring as natural a childbirth as possible, with minimal use of medical technology. These couples recognize the value of staying at home during the first part of labor but may not feel confident in being completely alone once the labor gets going. Fathers are often concerned, at first, that a birth assistant may somehow replace their role as the primary support person. They find out quickly, however, that a birth assistant helps ensure the sanctity of that role by handling the logistics surrounding the birth and by drawing on her experience to reassure and guide both father and mother through the natural challenges their birth will present to them.

> My doula was always on my side and I could count on her to support me in my decisions. I don't think I could have had an unmedicated birth without her.

One advantage of having a doula as birthing assistant instead of a family member or close friend is that the doula brings with her lots of experience. Another advantage is that you don't have to worry about how you are acting. With a doula, you are not distracted and can fully concentrate on the labor and birth.

There is just something extremely comforting about having an experienced woman there solely to help you.

Although you may think a doula is hired just to support the laboring woman, many partners say they valued their doula's presence tremendously, increasing their own confidence and their ability to be emotionally present with the laboring woman. When a couple has hired a doula, the partner doesn't have to remember everything he heard in childbirth class. Doulas encourage and support the partner's participation, recognizing how important the partner's support is to the future of the relationship and the health of the family. The doula is an invaluable resource in planning for birth, helping to assess the alignment of a provider and place of birth with the birth plan, being a knowledgeable and calming presence for the mother and partner from early contractions though birth and early breastfeeding.

> Our doula was invaluable in keeping both me and my husband calm when I started pushing before we left the house for our forty-five minute drive to the birth center. She rode with us in the truck on the way there and helped me remember to stay relaxed during contractions and helped him remain calm in between them, even when he turned onto the wrong side of the divided highway! I also found it really helpful to be physically reminded (by her laying her hands on my forehead) to keep relaxed, rather than being reminded vocally, and to never have to ask for water; before I even thought that I needed it, she was offering me my water bottle. —JEN BAJGER, mother of Diego, chose a doula for her first birth

Fathers benefit greatly from the presence of a doula. First of all, the doula can be given specific instructions to let the dad provide the comfort measures to the mom himself. The doula then can suggest the best comfort measures for the mom and can show the dad how to do them. If the doula weren't there, the dad might not remember all the massage techniques he learned in prenatal class. Another benefit for the dad is that while the doula massages the mom's back, for example, he can be face-to-face with his wife, holding her hands and providing words of support. If the mom is in more active labor and suddenly decides that no one should touch her, the doula can assure the surprised dad that this is normal in late labor and that he should not be offended or hurt.

Sometimes dads find it easier to follow instructions on how to comfort their wives rather than having to figure it out themselves, especially while they are worrying about the welfare of their partner and baby. A doula can help the dad deal with the mother during the difficult stage of transition, where moms often decide that they have had it with labor and may get discouraged. Without the doula there, the dad will feel pressured to take the pain away, although that is not what the mother is asking. Dads find that a doula can help them make sense of the situation. A doula can predict what the mom needs, allowing the dad to follow along or just be there for his wife emotionally. If he knows that the doula will take care of the physical support for the mom, he can concentrate on caressing her hair, giving her kisses, and saying words of support.

Women who labor with the help of a doula report feeling very satisfied with their husband's support and the birth experience overall. This is probably because the dad was encouraged to become involved in the labor by the presence of the doula.

~❧~

Is a doula an advocate?

Natural childbirth should definitely be more commonplace. The natural process of birth through hormonal changes prepares babies for transition outside the womb, facilitates bonding between mothers and babies, and prepares women for the tasks of motherhood. We need to make midwifery care widely available to birthing women, offering alternative options in childbirth education that reinforce the continuum between pregnancy, birth, and parenting. We also need to make emotional support and physical support for laboring women, or doula training, part of the education of medical and nursing students. Doula services need to be widely available and recognized for the very important and unique role that a doula offers a laboring woman. —TRACEY STOLARCHUK, doula, childbirth education instructor

A common misconception is that if you have a doctor who does not embrace natural childbirth, you can still have the natural birth you want by having a doula because she will be your advocate. The truth is that the most critical piece in the planning of a natural birth is the main caregiver, that is, the doctor or midwife. A doula can be your biggest ally, but she has no authority to dictate the course of your medical care; only you can do that. Even then, parents are often easily dissuaded from having a natural birth if their doctor does not prefer it.

A doula supports the mother in whatever birth plan or decisions she makes. The following is a pretty typical scenario of how a doula supports a mom in a hospital when the main caregiver wants to dramatically change the birth plan of a natural birth:

> The mom hires a doula because she wants a natural birth, after birthing her first child with vacuum and forceps. The mom chooses a new doctor this time because he is supportive of her birth plan.
>
> When labor begins, the mother labors calmly at home for a few hours with the doula. They use the bathtub, a birthing ball, and a back massage roller to cope with the contractions. The contractions get closer together until they are four minutes apart for over an hour. The father drives the car to the hospital while the doula rides in the back seat with the mom, supporting her during the contractions.
>
> At the hospital, the admission nurse checks the chart and learns that the mother had an epidural with her previous birth. She begins to follow the hospital's standard protocol for laboring moms: intravenous feed, continuous electronic fetal monitoring, and complete restriction of food. The mom looks at the doula in distress because this is exactly the sort of intervention she wanted to avoid. The doula smiles at her and asks her if she agrees to the procedures listed by the nurse. The mom says that she wants a natural birth. The nurse replies that she is only following hospital protocol. The mom says that she has a birth plan and that her doctor approved it. The nurse reads the birth plan and tells the mom that she will call the doctor and confirm the course of treatment.
>
> When the nurse leaves, the mom looks at her doula and asks her to intervene. The doula explains that the mom has control over her

own care and reminds her of all the items in her birth plan that included free mobility about the room and no intravenous feed. The nurse comes back with the doctor, and the doctor explains that she can have the natural birth she wants but that he recommends she stay on the monitor for at least twenty minutes and that she not eat, for he doesn't want her to throw up, which he says will make the intravenous feed necessary to keep her energy up. The mom looks at the doula again. The doula asks her if she agrees to have all these procedures or if she wants some time to think about it. The mom repeats that she wants a natural birth and that she specifically asked that there be no interventions. The doctor replies that he wants the best for her and her baby and that she can still have the natural birth she wanted but that he needs her to stay hydrated. The mother agrees. After all, it is just a needle in the arm and a monitor belt.

Laboring continues as the doula massages and reassures the mom that she is doing just fine. Later on, a different nurse checks on the mom and asks if she wants an epidural for the pain. The mom says she wants a natural birth. The nurse replies that this is fine but that an epidural will give her a chance to sleep. The mom looks at the doula, and the doula asks if she wants the epidural or if she wants some time to think about it. The mom says she needs time to think about it, and the nurse leaves. The doula suggests that they get in the shower and try some water relaxation.

After a shift change, a different nurse checks on the mom and offers her an epidural saying that she can see that the mom is really having a hard time during labor and that an epidural would give her a well-deserved rest. The mom is now having second thoughts but says no.

The doctor comes in to check on the mom and says that he is concerned that she has been laboring for a while now without a lot of improvement on the cervix dilation. He recommends that they start oxytocin to augment the labor. The mom looks at her doula, pleading with her to intervene. The doula asks the mom if she agrees to the procedure and reminds her that her birth plan included her wishes about not wanting oxytocin augmentation. The mom says that she is fine the way she is doing. The doctor replies that if labor goes on for too long, she might be too tired to push. The mom considers that the epidural will allow her to rest, so she says no to the oxytocin but agrees to the epidural.

The mom thinks that at this point she is more interested in avoiding the vacuum and the forceps than in having a natural birth. The doctor says that oxytocin augmentation is the standard procedure after an epidural because the epidural might slow down labor. She agrees to the oxytocin too.

Eventually, the mom avoids the forceps and vacuum and births vaginally. The baby is in great health, but the mom has some complications from the epidural causing her to stay in the hospital an extra day for observation. She did not have a natural birth, but she felt satisfied that she at least gave it a try. She wished the doula had told the nurses to stop suggesting the epidural.

We see that the doula did everything she told the mom she would do: she offered her massage, advised her to change positions, and provided emotional support. But when it came to making decisions about medical care, the mom had to agree or disagree to the proposed procedures. It is important to remember then that a doula will help remind you and your partner of your birth plans and alternatives, but she will not speak on your behalf. The doula can only do so much in an environment that she doesn't control. If the parents are convinced that they want to have a natural birth, having a doula can keep them on track with their birth plan and provide the comfort needed by the mother to immerse herself in labor and relax enough to allow the contractions to work.

A misconception is that doulas are completely nonpartisan when caring for their clients. A happy mother doesn't always a happy doula make. Doulas will do what the mothers ask of them but certainly recommend natural childbirth options. When you meet with a specific birth assistant, tell her about the kind of birth you want and about any prior birth experiences, including any differences you would like to see from your last birth. A doula will also screen her clients to ensure proper fit with parents who match her view of birth. Most doulas support natural birth as a matter of principle, since the majority of their training is on natural alternatives to obstetrical intervention.

During doula training, students are often asked to consider what kind of advocate they are or will become: an advocate for the mother, an advocate for the baby, or an advocate for the method of birth. A doula who feels her job is to advocate for the mother will support any decision the mother makes and will suggest comfort measures that will make the mother comfortable, even if that means deviating from the planned birth method or if the benefits to the baby are questionable; for example, offering an epidural to take all the pain away from the mom increases the chances of caesarean and possibly passes medication into the baby's bloodstream. On the other hand, a doula may feel that her job is to advocate for the baby, meaning that she will strive to offer the mom comfort measures and labor enhancing measures that can ensure the baby's welfare but may not completely satisfy the mom or follow the planned method of birth, such as pushing the mom into an upright position to prevent the baby from getting stuck but causing the mom to get up from the bed when she doesn't want to do so. Finally, a doula who feels she is an advocate for the method of birth might concentrate her efforts on avoiding a caesarean, for example, rather than try to provide complete comfort for the mother or considering whether the baby can handle a long labor.

In all these cases, it's important to remember that doulas will support you in whatever course of treatment you choose. After all, your body is the one receiving the treatment. If your doula is an advocate for natural birth and you know you want one and are prepared to work hard for it, then the odds are that the birth will go as planned, making both of you happy. But if you know that the moment you walk into the hospital, you will be getting drugs and an epidural, tell this to the doula. It would be better to be honest with your doula and allow her to be selective in the clients she accepts. She will still be prepared to give you options of care, including answering your questions about epidurals and referring you to other doulas.

Ask your doula what types of births she has witnessed: caesarean, epidural, intervention free, vaginal birth after caesarean, teen birth, and so on. This can help you avoid the pitfalls she has seen occur in other births. Ask her if she has ever worked with your care provider or at your place of birth. This can help you predict the course of this provider's care.

Avoiding the wrong doula is also an important part of preparing for a natural birth. Find out if the doula is affiliated with the hospital in which you plan to give birth. If she is, then it is possible that she may try hard to cooperate with the hospital staff at the expense of her commitment to support you.

Talking to a doula's previous clients can help you select one based on her experience, her attitude, and her quirks. It's a good idea to meet a few doulas before hiring one, to compare and contrast, noting with whom you find yourself feeling most comfortable for this blessed event in your lives. Doulas vary in experience, specialty, fees, and styles.

> Well, she said she absolutely did not want anyone at this birth to tell her to shut up and stay in control. She said the feeling in her was so wild. She didn't know what it was, but she wanted to do as she pleased at this birth. All she wanted me to do was just be her guardian, to watch over the safety of her and her baby as the baby was being born. So I agreed to her wishes.

~∾∽

Do I need a doula if I already have a midwife?

It is a common myth among midwifery clients that because the woman has a midwife, she no longer needs to have a doula. In fact, midwives and doulas are quite a team. The doula can be present supporting the laboring woman for many hours before there is a need to call the midwife. This is particularly true of home births. Doulas are especially helpful when the midwife is attending another birth and will be delayed. At the moment of birth, the midwife will understandably concentrate on the baby, leaving the doula to focus exclusively on the needs of the mother. During potentially traumatic births when the midwife needs to focus on medical procedures, having a doula can guarantee that the woman will receive continuous emotional support and attention. The value of having a doula available is especially critical during and after caesareans because the physical and emotional needs of the woman have not changed, and in fact they may be greater.

A phenomenon now developing is the use of doulas every time a woman or man enters the hospital for medical treatment, surgery, or terminal care. The need for continuous and dedicated support during these potentially stressful events seems obvious. The doula can be a private advocate and a consultant to guide the educated consumer through the bureaucratic maze that hospital care can be. As mentioned before, in these situations the emotional and physical needs of the person may be great.

Choosing a supportive caregiver, be it a physician or a midwife, is the most critical step toward achieving natural birth. But having a doula is the icing on the cake of a woman's natural birth plan. The doula offers dedicated labor support from even before labor starts to some time after the baby is born. All this support is in addition to the medical care provided by the physician and the midwife throughout the whole prenatal and postnatal phase.

CLAUDIA (GÓMEZ) VILLENEUVE was born in Barranquilla, Colombia, and moved to Canada in 1992. She graduated from civil engineering school with a master's in construction management from the University of Alberta. Her first child was born by nonemergency caesarean after a failed induction. When she became pregnant with her second child, she planned to have a vaginal birth after caesarean (VBAC). Her successful home water birth with a midwife gave her the inspiration to take the DONA (Doulas of North America) training and become a doula. She lectures on caesarean avoidance and has published related articles for various English- and Spanish-speaking publications. Her birth stories are <www.edmontonVBAC.netfirms.com>.

PAM SOROCHAN'S BIRTH STORY

I did not believe because I could not see.
When the dawn seemed forever lost,
You showed me your love in the light of the stars.
Then the mountain rose before me,
By the deep well of desire,
From the fountain of forgiveness,
Beyond the ice and the fire.
Give these clay feet wings to fly
To touch the face of the stars.
Breathe life into this feeble heart
Lift this mortal veil of fear
Take these crumbled hopes, etched with tears
We'll rise above these earthly cares.

—*Dante's Prayer*, Loreena McKennitt

WHEN KYNAN WAS born on December twenty-sixth by caesarean section, I
was stunned. When I think of it now, I can still hardly believe it had happened
to me. I was a registered nurse at the time, and I trusted the hospital to take care
of me. I did everything they said, I read all my textbooks, and still it happened
to me. My baby was fine, and after a while so was I, physically. I've heard it said
that we have to heal physically before our minds and spirits will be ready. I
remember the time that I began to realize that things might not have needed
to happen the way they did. I was convinced that I must have missed something.
I have cried about not getting to see my precious little son be born. I am sad-
dened by waking from anesthesia and not remembering I had had a baby. I
longed for that experience of birthing a baby. I began a quest to find out if things
could be different next time, if I could brave a next time.

My husband's unfailing ear as he listened helped me heal, and the local
VBAC group was my greatest source of hope. I was suddenly surrounded by

women, options, and alternatives that thrilled me. I read and asked questions and listened to many wise words. I learned not to feel guilty, I learned not to blame myself, and I learned not to be afraid. I decided that, unlike last time, I couldn't go into this labor just expecting I would know what to do and expecting someone else to get me through it. I learned of the power of my body and my mind and my will. I learned that these tiny lives inside are not just passive participants in this beautiful journey.

When we were finally pregnant again, Mike and I discussed a home birth. I spoke with some wonderful midwives and friends and felt very intrigued with the idea. Because of the emergency experience of our first birth, Mike said he felt safest in the hospital in case anything happened. In the journey of birthing our children, I would be fine in the hospital, so we made our plans to go there.

> I just want to be understood and for things to go my way. I've decided that it is not the doctor who will make this happen but me.
> —June twenty-second, 17 weeks

> I hate terms like "trial of labor" and "a good chance that you'll…" They are so ambiguous and noncommittal. I'm looking for cheerleaders. —July twentieth, 21 weeks

This time I was grateful for my medical background in a different way. I was aware of doctors' strengths and weaknesses. I don't like how most doctors treat pregnant women, as if they have an illness and as if pregnancy is all about the body and has nothing to do with the mind. I was lucky to find an obstetrician who would support me in my endeavors but soon felt that he was more of a formality than a necessity. I found a gifted doula who believed in me and pushed away any remaining doubts and fears. I deeply wanted to do this without any interference. My thoughts were that the longer I spent at the hospital and the more they interfered, the greater the chance that things would go wrong. I wanted to labor at home and find natural ways for comfort and relief during labor.

> Sometimes I'm so excited and entranced about this baby coming, and sometimes I'm so scared about how it will be.
> —August twenty-eight, 27 weeks

As I visualized the birth of my baby, the head would stop right before it came out, right where my son's head had stopped during my first birth. I spent a lot of time trying to connect my body and mind and to resolve the fears that would surface there. I'm not sure anyone knows how scared I was that this might not happen. Even now I look at the large tree full of leaves blowing in the wind outside our back window and remember the music I chose that would give me strength and power, the relaxation that would give me relief, and the visualizations that would conquer the barriers of my mind.

> We met with our doula again on Friday. I feel very confident with my little support team. —September twenty-six, 31 weeks

Eleven days before Anna's due date, at about eight AM, I started feeling cramps. I felt it couldn't possibly be labor because it was too early, so I continued about my day, even taking Kynan to gymnastics and participating in floor games there as my cramps grew worse. Over the previous couple of weeks, the baby's movements had decreased a bit, so I was booked for a nonstress test at the hospital at ten forty-five AM. As I dropped Kynan off before my test, a little voice told me that I would not be back for him that day. I laugh now at how I pushed that thought aside, not wanting to make something out of nothing.

My mild discomfort and the fetal heart monitor on my huge belly told me that I was indeed in labor. I didn't feel ready for this, and at noon I tearfully phoned Mike to join me. "Is home really where you think you should be if you're in labor?" a nurse said.

"If this is going to be a long labor, I'm going to go home."

At about one PM, my contractions became regular and close but were still tolerable. I was anticipating many hours of labor—my first was fifteen and a half hours—and I had planned on laboring at home. But as my discomfort quickly increased, the voice inside seemed to tell me to stay at the hospital, and I finally listened to it. With my first child so much of my labor had frightened me, and my labor had been very different from the textbook labors I had read about. But with this labor it all seemed familiar somehow and even reassuring, knowing that my body had done these same things before. This time I was no longer afraid. This was my body, my labor, and my way.

At about one thirty PM, my contractions exploded, and I knew we were on our way. After that I had no concept of time. The contractions were powerful, with no time to rest in between, and the shower brought no relief. As I left the shower to head for the tub room (I think neither midwives nor laboring women designed hospital facilities!), I was confronted with the hospital's routine procedure of rupturing the membranes. I didn't even give them time to ask me or take that little plastic hook out of the package: as soon as I saw it, I said I didn't want it done. The doctor had no problem with my refusal; the nurse seemed put out. Next an epidural and medication were offered; I refused them, too. (It makes me wonder how many women actually get past three centimeters before their strength is undermined and they succumb to drugs.) The big tub was a little better. I had Mike call for our doula to come. The contractions were furious, and Mike kept trying to help me relax and remind me that this was pain with a purpose. I wanted a break from the pain so badly.

Many tearful prayers had petitioned the granting of a beautiful birth for me, and I believe our prayers are answered in unique and wonderful ways. Because of my haste in the morning, I didn't have my prenatal records or birth plan with me, and my obstetrician was on vacation, so it had not been revealed that I was having a vaginal birth after caesarean. When the nurse stormed into the tub room demanding to know why I hadn't told her I was a VBAC, she wanted me to get out of the tub and "safely" into bed and be strapped to equipment immediately. I briefly explained my understanding of her concerns and stated that I didn't plan on going anywhere.

Finally our doula came, and it was like a cool refreshing breeze floated into the room. She dimmed the lights and guided me through ways to get myself coping again. With my first labor I was very concerned with how far apart the contractions were and how long I'd been in labor and how dilated I was. Now I was just thrilled to be doing it and was too busy to think about any of that. Then as I breathed out, I felt a mild urge to push. The nurse wouldn't check my cervix in the tub. As I got out, I felt my water break. The labor was so intense that I didn't care where I was anymore. Walking just made one big, long contraction. My cervix was dilated eight centimeters, they said. "Already!" I thought.

The pressure on my perineum was unreal. When I came out of the bathroom, the nurse announced that she wanted to put in an intravenous feed. With genuine amazement I asked, "Why do I need an IV?!" "Because you're a VBAC!" "I don't want an IV!" And I didn't have one.

I knelt by the bed for a while. I didn't think about anyone else but my baby and myself. As much as it hurt, it seemed so natural and all just flowed from me. Mike gave me his strength, and our doula gave me focus and purpose. Eventually, I ended up on the bed. I hadn't imagined that the pain would be continuous. People have spoken of the overpowering urge to push, and I always wondered what it would feel like. Then suddenly it was there, and it was amazing! Since my cervix wasn't quite ready yet, I had to breath through this uncontrollable urge. I think this was harder than the whole rest of labor. Several times I couldn't stop myself from pushing. It felt so good! Then nothing could stop me, and I was told to go ahead. Then they wanted me to wait for the doctor but I didn't. "I love pushing!"

It's all so much more wonderful and powerful and painful than I thought it would be. No one's counting and telling me to push because I can't feel the contractions, no one's watching a heart rate drop on a monitor, no one's shaving my hair, no one's telling me to sign forms I haven't read, and I'm feeling everything!

> I scream and her head is out. Oh, it hurts, and her body is out. It's
> 4:28 PM, November 12. Everyone else seems to disappear, and it's just
> me and Mike and our girl.

The pain ended so suddenly. I am so grateful for the success of her birth and how much joy and love there was. I waited so long for that moment of seeing one of my babies be born. All my babies will have come into this world in a different way. Kynan's birth changed my life and created the motivation for the amazing event of Anna's birth.

࣮

VALERIE LARENNE'S BIRTH STORY

BEFORE I BECAME pregnant for the first time, I thought natural childbirth was for granola-bar hippie types at best or fanatical masochists at worst. It was most certainly not for me, a modern woman of the twenty-first century. I never once questioned whether or not I would have an epidural if I were to be so lucky as to get pregnant. Like a lot of women, I envisioned walking into the hospital the day I was due and screaming, "Give me drugs, now!" After all, everyone I knew who had had a baby had had an epidural. Why not take advantage of the wonderful tools available to us now through the miracle of modern medicine? Case closed, slam-dunk, right?

Well, as it turned out, the day I found out I was pregnant was also the day that my eyes began to open about the realities of childbirth. It soon became clear to me that the medical establishment in which I had placed such blind faith was not necessarily treating my pregnant self with my own and my baby's best interests in mind. I am not saying that the medical establishment intended me any harm per se; rather, I think the traditional obstetrical model has become so burdened by the threat of costly litigation and so hamstrung by the insurance industry that it has been forced to manage childbirth and mold it to serve the needs of the medical establishment, not the needs of women. If I could shout to the rooftops so all pregnant women could hear, I would tell them, "You are stronger than you think, you can have your birth your way, and birth is something to anticipate with joy, not something to dread and fear."

I started my journey down the commonly trod path, straight to the best obstetrician I could find in my area. At only ten weeks, we had an internal ultrasound and heard a heart beating, and I thought I would burst with joy. I had been trying for so long to have a baby that I was beginning to wonder if I would ever be able to conceive. Here was proof, right there on that gray monitor with that ocean-like whooshing sound, that I was going to become a mommy.

But this was also when I started to see that the journey I had embarked upon was not what I was expecting. Because I was thirty-five when I found out I was pregnant, I fell into a category called advanced maternal age. The first choice I was then forced to make was whether or not to have an amniocentesis. I carefully read the literature and discovered that I had a greater chance of having a miscarriage from the procedure than I did of carrying a sick baby, so I promptly opted out. I also learned that higher resolution ultrasounds are able to detect a wide range of abnormalities. Best of all, they are totally noninvasive. I had a higher resolution ultrasound at twenty weeks, and it put my mind completely at ease about the health of my baby.

I was already becoming very protective of my baby and less confident that the doctor was interested in what I had in mind for my birthing. With each visit to this "expert," my sense of unease grew. He seemed dismissive of me in general and cautioned me not to talk to my mother or girlfriends about any questions or concerns I had. With a wink and a smile he said, "If you have a question, talk to me. When you start talking to other people, you'll just get confused." "Hmmm," I thought, "Really? Do I look that stupid to you?" Clearly this was not a good sign. I thought my growing discomfort had to do with the fact that my doctor was a man. "Shame on me," I thought, "I'm just so used to my female doctor that I can't relate to this guy. Surely if I have a female obstetrician, I'll feel much better." So I sheepishly asked for a change of doctors and was excited the day I was to meet with my new female obstetrician.

Prior to meeting the new obstetrician, I had been reading books about childbirth. The most valuable of these was *Birthing from Within* by Pam England and Rob Horowitz. This book caused a revolution in my thinking about birthing. I learned all sorts of things that doctors never tell you about what it means to choose a medicated birth, including that in most cases it's not even a choice. I learned that if you go into your birthing experience without any knowledge about the process, you are completely vulnerable to what the hospital and doctors have in mind for you.

Every pregnant woman owes it to herself and her baby to become educated so she can make an informed choice. There is a lack of balanced information available to women from their doctors. Believe me when I say that they are trying to do what is convenient and less potentially litigious for them. They are not necessarily in business to advocate for their patients, especially when what their patient wants does not fit the standard model.

Don't ever forget: you are hiring the doctor, not the other way around. You have the power to set the agenda for your birth. If you feel that your caregiver is not letting you set the agenda, then you need to find another caregiver. This is very important.

It has been my experience that a midwife is far better than an obstetrician for a pregnant woman. This choice is a no-brainer as far as I'm concerned. Babies are born by women, not delivered by doctors. (Pizzas are delivered, not babies.) Midwives view pregnancy and birth as the most natural aspects of womanhood and treat you more like a very special person who happens to be pregnant than just another patient who needs to be cured. Compared to doctors, midwives have much lower rates of episiotomies, epidurals, and caesarean sections. Midwives are with the birthing mother during the entire birthing process, unlike most obstetricians, who leave the real work to the nurses during a woman's birthing time only to show up at the last minute to catch the baby.

This brings me back to my experience with the new doctor that I was excited about. Unfortunately, she was even worse than the male obstetrician. I could not imagine this woman in the delivery room dealing with all the blood and fluids involved in birthing a baby. When I started going over my list of questions, she was visibly annoyed. When I asked her, "How will you support me in my desire for a natural birth?" she looked at me like I had just landed from the planet Mars and instead of answering my question, she said, "Well, you wouldn't have a filling in your tooth done without Novocain, now, would you?" Aside from the fact that this analogy was totally irrelevant, her being dismissive of my desires was all I needed to know to take my body and my baby out the door. That was when this mama began her search for a midwife in earnest.

Luckily, there are a few enlightened hospitals within comfortable driving distance from me that allow midwife-assisted births. The place where I ended up birthing my son was fabulous, very supportive of natural approaches to birth and providing much more individualized care, with a monthly average of around sixty births compared to well over 400 at some busy hospitals. In addition, their birthing rooms are labor-delivery-recovery (LDR), and they have a rooming-in policy for newborns.

In addition to finding a supportive team of midwives, I was eager to take a birthing course that would help me have the natural birth I had now come to desire so strongly. I looked into a program called Hypnobabies, which sounds a lot wackier than it is. It is a program that teaches a woman how to go into a state of self-induced hypnosis to assist during her birthing and develop the skills necessary to tap into the body's natural well of pain management chemicals. Anyone can do it; it's just a matter of desire and commitment. I can't tell you how many times I have heard women (me included) say, "I'm pretty tough, and I'd like to do it naturally, so I'll just go to the hospital and see how it goes." But that is about as smart as saying, "I think I'd like to climb Mount Everest, so I'm going to take the first plane I can find to Nepal and see how it goes." Any difficult physical task such as running a marathon or giving birth requires preparation, both physical and mental. Natural birthing courses such as the Bradley method and Hypnobabies provide this necessary training.

I practiced my self-hypnosis daily and did everything I could to surround myself with nothing but positive birth imagery. During this process I became very excited about the impending birth of my son. As I got closer and closer to my due date, people asked me, "Are you getting nervous yet?" I could honestly say that I was not nervous but happy about my upcoming birthing and in a state of hopeful curiosity.

About a week and a half before my son was due to arrive, I awoke at six AM, and as I was getting out of bed, I felt as if a bubble burst and a little gush of liquid ran out of me. I had always thought of my water breaking as more like Niagara Falls, so I wasn't sure if what I had felt was my water breaking or a little "accident." Something about it just didn't feel right, though, so I called my midwife to say that I thought my water had broken. Sure enough, the Niagara Falls effect occurred shortly thereafter, so there was no doubt in my mind that this was the day.

My husband and I spent it in a sort of twilight zone, as there were no significant contractions. I visited my midwife at noon to discover that I was only half a centimeter dilated and fifty percent effaced. We agreed to meet at the hospital at six o'clock that night, and she explained that we would have to consider Pitocin between midnight and two AM if no further progress had been made.

Prior to my son's birth, we had hired a doula trained in the Hypnobabies process to assist us. Carole arrived at our home about an hour before we needed to leave for the hospital. She brought with her a special hypnosis script to help release my mind from anything that was holding my body back from starting my birthing time. It was an incredible experience. I felt as if all the molecules in my body melted away, and I entered a deep state of relaxation. During our drive to the hospital I listened to the Birth Guide CD from my Hypnobabies class with my eyes closed. Our arrival at the hospital was relaxed, peaceful, and stress free.

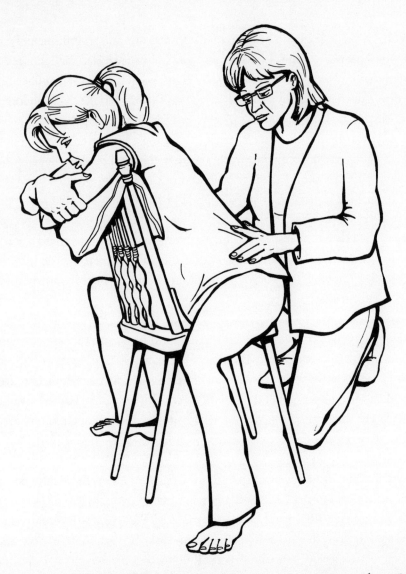

Sitting backward on a chair while getting a LOWER BACK MASSAGE is a popular position in labor. A cushion can be wedged below the woman's buttocks to lift her and tilt the uterus forward, which aids in optimal positioning of the baby. Tilting the uterus backward, such as lying on your back in a bed, has two undesirable consequences: one, the weight of baby and uterus press on the vena cava, a major vein that provides oxygen to the placenta and the baby; and two, the baby's weight shifts away from the cervix, where the pressure is needed, and to the woman's spine, increasing her pain. Some massage is helpful in easing the pain of the contractions, and since most women feel them in the lower part of the back, that is where massaging by the labor support person can be most effective. The massage can extend to the shoulders, where a lot of stress is collected, and then down on either side of the spine to the base.

Once I was admitted, my midwife administered a prostaglandin suppository to help ripen the cervix. Still, progress was slow in coming. When it seemed that nothing much would happen that night, my parents left to go home to sleep, and our doula went with them, as she needed to go back to pick up her car. Like magic, the minute the people who were waiting, waiting, waiting for me to have the baby left the scene, my birthing waves began in earnest. It seemed like my body needed to be in a little cocoon with just my husband and me in order to get truly ready for the birth of our son.

My birthing time began at around ten-thirty that night and lasted until four forty-five the following morning when our son Jordan was born. For a first pregnancy this was fairly short, and the time-compression phenomenon common in hypnosis made those six hours feel like even less. During that time my doula, midwife, and husband helped me through each birthing wave with a variety of measures such as showering, changing positions, rocking on the birthing ball, applying warm back compresses, using gentle massage, using scented fans, and offering soothing words that helped me stay deeply relaxed throughout each one. I recall only quiet, loving words and caresses. My eyes were closed almost the entire time, and I had the feeling of being in a soft, safe place.

My own method of coping with the waves came from deep within, something not practiced in the class and something that I can only describe as primal. With each wave I found that I would instinctively hum. There was something very soothing about certain tonal sounds, and I varied these with each wave until I hit the right note to get through to the end. As a regular practitioner of yoga I also found the "om" sound helpful. I recall feeling intense pressure, but not pain in the traditional sense of the word. One of the most helpful things about this time was not constantly being told how far I was progressing. The only time I was told how far I had dilated was when I was at seven and a half centimeters, and I remember thinking, "Well, if I've gone this far without needing anything for my discomfort, I can certainly go all the way!" The only other progress report I received was when I was at nine and a half centimeters.

The pushing phase of labor lasted approximately an hour and a half and was the most difficult part of the journey. It was frustrating at times in being physically exhausting, like running a marathon, but not painful. I recall the soothing sensation of warm compresses but no pain. I recall Carole repeating these words to me, "Your body is sending anesthesia ahead of your baby." Clearly, my body was doing this. I had no feelings of discomfort when my midwife reached in to help fully open my cervix. I had no feelings of discomfort when my son crowned. There was no ring of fire. Nothing. The only discomfort I experienced during this time was the work my abdomen was doing to help push the baby out, kind of like overdoing it on the ab machine at the gym.

When my son was born, he was placed immediately into my hands and I brought him up to my chest. It is a moment I will never forget. His bright little eyes were sparkling, and he took to my breast within minutes. He was alert and very much engaged in the world. From the moment of his birth I felt absolutely nothing but pure joy. All the frustration of the pushing phase vanished, and I was giggling. There was no pain in my body. I had a minor tear that was quickly and painlessly repaired (also without anesthetic), and from that moment I did not need anything for pain because I did not feel any pain.

I'm living proof that it's true: you can give birth without so much as an aspirin. I did it thanks to the loving support of a trained doula and midwife, a supportive and engaged partner, and the mental tools that I developed through practice to have the birthing experience I wanted. The biggest gift I feel that I gave to myself and to my son in this process was being fully present in both mind and body for the incredible experience of his birthing. There are times when I worry that my desire to share the tale of my son's birthing verges on religious zeal, but when I hear women who have been so sadly disappointed by their less-than-empowering births, I want every woman to have the opportunity to experience the kind of birthing that I did.

Barb Silvestro's birth story

Both my girls were born by emergency caesarean surgeries. The first birth occurred when I was twenty-four years old and knew nothing. Honestly, I knew nothing. I did what my doctors told me. When my water began to leak, I dutifully went to the hospital. I was induced with Pitocin, took Demerol, and when the baby went into distress after an hour of pushing, we had emergency surgery.

After divorce and then remarriage nine years afterward, I became pregnant and started researching vaginal birth after caesarean. I read a bit but not nearly as much as I should have. I was thirty-five years old and very nervous about labor and birth. When my doctor suggested we induce at thirty-eight weeks because the baby was getting very big, I agreed. I was induced with Pitocin, had an epidural, and guess what? The baby went into distress and off we went for a caesarean birth.

My girls are both healthy and happy at ages thirteen (Chelsey) and three (Zoey). But when we discovered my pregnancy with this baby, our last, I was bound and determined to have him naturally. No interventions, no surgery.

I read and read and read. I talked with other mamas. I found a midwife to work with who supported my decision for a natural vaginal birth after caesarean. I read on the Internet, and at the library. I read birth stories. I prayed. I meditated. I practiced squatting and moving and moaning. I worked on my feelings about birthing in the hospital since the birthing center wouldn't allow vaginal births after caesareans there and my husband was too upset by the last birth experience to be comfortable with home birth. We talked about staying home until I was sure it was active labor. We had a birth plan and knew what we wanted.

Finally it was time. I was thirty-seven weeks and six days into the pregnancy and had been having what I thought were some sporadic Braxton Hicks contractions the last few days, not increasing in frequency, not increasing in intensity.

I took my three-year-old and the twenty-month-old that I babysit to playgroup and ate cupcakes that my friend had made for my birthday, which was coming up that weekend. Then home for the afternoon, nothing too exciting. We ate a nice dinner and went for a swim. After that I dried off and lay down in bed to do a hypnobirthing relaxation tape. Suddenly I felt a popping and rolled out of the bed just as I started to gush. It was eight forty PM, and my water had broken.

I figured we had plenty of time, since no real contractions had started, so we puttered around for a bit, packing the bag, getting stuff into coolers, etc. I jumped online to let folks know what was happening and to e-mail my friend Darshani, who was going to be our labor support person/doula. Everyone pretty much agreed that it was still early: I should take a shower, listen to more hypnobirthing tapes, try to rest.

I tried, but my body had other ideas. I started contracting harder and faster. I called Darshani at ten PM, when I couldn't talk through the contractions, which were coming four to five minutes apart. By the time she arrived at eleven PM, the shower didn't help, the hypnobirthing tapes had been tossed, and I was being extremely vocal about the intensity of contractions and how much they sucked. After I had three contractions two to three minutes apart lasting fifty-five to sixty seconds and telling her, "I think I might get an epidural after all," we all decided it was time to go to the hospital.

We drove downtown while I experienced fierce contractions. The exit ramp to the hospital was blocked off for construction, but luckily the next exit was open so we got there by eleven twenty. The nurse checked me, and I was dilated to four to five centimeters if she stretched me. I almost died. I told them, "The hell with it. They're too close together, too strong, and I'm only at four to five?? Get me an epidural." My doula talked to me about how I was doing so well and stalled the anesthesiologist—good woman, that doula.

About fifteen to twenty minutes went by, with contractions so hard and fast I couldn't walk, squat, or move. I just hung on to the bed rail for dear life and did hard breathing—heeeeee heeeeeeee hooooooo—and low moans. I cussed a few times, too, telling them it had to stop and to get the **** anesthesiologist. I probably screamed as well, but my support team was amazing. (Darshani says I didn't scream, but I don't believe her.)

The anesthesiologist finally did show up, but it was too late, as I was telling them that I needed to push. I was shaking, and I remember Darshani telling me that I was in transition: the baby was almost here. The nurse checked me, and I was eight to nine centimeters dilated with a bit of a lip. She told me she was going to push the lip aside and have me push. I pushed through the lip to ten and moved him down, she said afterward, two inches or so, and she said, "Okay, stop. I feel his noggin; we need to get the midwife." I looked up at Tom and told him, "Go get Chelsey, now." He looked at me like I was nuts, and I reminded him that I had promised her she wouldn't miss it.

I yelled over to the midwife, "He's coming on the next push." Darshani says it was only one big push, but I think it was really three, and he was out. He was born at 12:54 AM, four and a half hours after labor started. He weighed in at seven pounds, two ounces and was nineteen and a half inches long.

The midwife put him on my chest, and they wiped him down. I just couldn't stop looking at him and crying. After the cord stopped pulsing, big sister Chelsey cut it, a big moment for her. He honestly looked like a truck had hit him. He was purple, and his eyes were swollen and bugged out and bloodshot. But he was still so cute, with his big eyes and so much hair. His Apgars were eight and nine, even with the trauma of such a quick birth. He nursed immediately and got pink right away. The hospital staff totally respected all our wishes. No one took him until I gave them permission to weigh him—right next to me in the room—then they left us alone. It was wonderful. I did get a few looks when I said no to some of the routine things they do, but they respected our wishes and left us alone with our son.

After everyone held him and we took a zillion pictures, I sent everyone home and he and I cuddled, nursed, and slept for a few hours. I have to say that after the caesarean births, the recovery was easy. I was walking, eating, talking, playing. The uterine contractions/cramps were sometimes pretty heavy, but much easier to deal with than stomach surgery.

I had a wonderful experience with vaginal birth after caesarean. Only thing that could've been better was if it had been just a little slower.

Our son's name is Roman Thomas Silvestro. We're calling him Romy for short since Roman is a big name for such a small boy. That's my story. A hospital birth, but natural; a vaginal birth after two caesareans, by a thirty-eight-year-old mama. Not bad, eh?

Dana (Ksenia) Ovcharenko's birth story

At the age of thirty-seven, I gave birth to my first child in Kiev, Ukraine, where I had been living for six years. The pregnancy was exhilarating, and I blithely battled the post-Soviet medical system, which was bound and determined to make me into a sick person, frowning disapprovingly on my steady weight gain and insisting that I should be hospitalized for my swollen ankles. I was far from home and did not have the benefit of prenatal classes, but I had lots of literature and used the Internet as an information resource, and I was quite confident that I was as informed as need be for the upcoming big event. As it turned out, of course, I was wholly unprepared for the birth itself. Even the fact that I was overdue, I now suspect, was my little one graciously hanging in there as long as she could while her mother tried to wrap her mind around this huge life-changing event, helpless as a deer caught in the beam of approaching headlights. Panic? No. Just the numb bewilderment of the modern woman, used to controlling everything around her, forced to face the unknown and uncontrollable and lacking the experience or faith to deal with it properly. So, yeah, I guess it was panic, the quiet, foggy panic of ignorance and denial.

Finally Maria could wait no more, and one morning I woke up and let go water that was black with meconium. The only reason I was not in the hospital and induced already was that my husband was a doctor, albeit in an unrelated specialty, which was sufficient in terms of clout to allow me to stay away until the last moment.

We drove to the maternity hospital where I had made prior arrangements. (The system was set up such that pregnancies were monitored locally by obstetrician-gynecologists while births were handled by obstetrical surgeons who only worked in the maternity hospitals.) I was given an enema. I wanted to move around, but they laughed and made me lie down when I instinctively moved into an all-fours position. I saw epidurals being administered, and on the whole I had every confidence in the medical skills of the personnel. But I wasn't dilating (not at all surprising, now that I consider it), they didn't want to wait because of the meconium, and of course they were understandably nervous about their naïve foreign client with the medical spouse.

Thus, I was prevailed upon to agree to a caesarean. It was a bikini-line incision done under general anesthesia, and my daughter of 10.3 pounds was born.

I recovered quickly and extremely well and was allowed to visit Maria in the neonatal intensive care unit, where she contrasted noticeably with all the preemies. On the third day they gave her to me in my private room, all swaddled in the Slavic style, and she stayed with me around the clock from then on, sleeping a good three to four hours at a stretch and breastfeeding without a hitch. We were discharged on the seventh day.

To this part of the story I want to add an unexpected, life-changing occurrence. By some miracle a copy of *The Continuum Concept* by Jean Liedloff that my sister had sent me from North America was delivered to my bedside in Kiev on the day after I gave birth, and I read most of it during that week. I was appalled by the descriptions of the isolation and abandonment felt by infants from their point of view, even though their parents may think the babies are getting the best of care. I wept for my own infancy and vowed to bring up my babies following the principles of attachment parenting. (This I have done, nursing my first well into my second pregnancy and co-sleeping as well.)

Caesarean birth is major abdominal surgery, often the result of a cascade of medical interventions. The term seems to me very apt because the consequences of one intervention (induction, epidural, even being forced to lie down in bed while laboring) often necessitate the next, and lead to an inevitable conclusion. It was not interventions per se that led to my first child being born by caesarean. I see now that our upbringing as modern women (read: control freaks) makes childbirth intimidating and, especially during the process, frightening because we do not have any experience with it. This fear, combined with the strong consumerist tendency in Western culture to avoid pain, completely eliminates the possibility for us to remain calm in the face of the unknown and have the faith to handle it. This is where I have become convinced that doulas have an important role to play.

———

WHEN I BECAME pregnant a second time, my first child was twenty-seven months old. I decided to move back home and chose to settle in the city of my high school years. Here the story becomes more ordinary in some ways (obstetrician, prenatal classes, etc.), but again I felt pressure from the medical system because I had had a caesarean section. In addition, I had no choice about my doctor because I arrived five months pregnant and had to take what I could get. After attending a meeting of a VBAC (vaginal birth after caesarean) association, I was inspired to hire a doula, and I also enlisted the support of a close friend whose second child was born with a vaginal birth after caesarean at home. She lent me her copy of *Open Season,* which I read avidly, and for the first time looked back at my caesarean as something other than the necessity I had always believed it was.

Thus armed, I was able to insist that I wanted to try a vaginal birth after cae-sarean and without pain medication. I also got the obstetrician's agreement to let me stay at home for the first part of labor and that I would not be put on an intravenous drip once I checked into the hospital (just a Hep lock), significant concessions given my high-risk category (VBAC plus age). I had gained a ton, going from 155 to over 220 pounds. I had huge, um, appetites that were just not being satisfied. But the baby seemed to be within normal limits. (I knew from the ultrasounds in Kiev before we moved back that it was a girl.) Not having to worry as much about the motherhood part of it the second time round, I was even more aware and therefore perhaps more apprehensive about the unknown quality of this birth, but this time I also had help, and that was my saving grace.

I was barely a week overdue but right on schedule given my extended cycle and my knowledge of the exact conception date. Regular contractions began at ten PM, and for the next two hours I continued to work on my computer at home. At midnight I felt a distinct pop in my belly, as though Sofia had a cro-chet hook inside, and my water let go. It was also stained with meconium but much more faintly, it seemed, than three years before. In any case, we drove to the hospital right away, and by the time I checked in, the contractions were com-ing every three minutes. All my careful plans (music, counting angels in my life, prayer) went out the window as things accelerated very rapidly. I was fright-ened by the labor pains as they approached. There is no way I could have made it through them without the doula Tracey and my friend Lorene, who held my hands, kept my eyes focused on theirs, and reassured me constantly that I was doing great. Moreover, the birth plan that the doula had taken the trouble to make with us ahead of time recalled the forgotten option of Entonox (50 percent oxygen, 50 percent nitrous oxide), which was blessedly effective and the only medication I used.

It was—I can now say—fantastic. I was rampant in the labor room, totally naked and howling. The doctor insisted on putting a scalp monitor on the baby, which was the undoing of his scheming interventions because I heard Sofia's heartbeat through it all and it was steady and strong. By five AM I was in transition and could not believe my ears when the doula told me that the doctor had announced that he would use suction. I shouted, "No!" The doctor was miffed, but his nurse was excellent. She helped very ably to direct my breathing and pushing, though I didn't follow her one hundred percent; I also listened to my own instincts.

The moment when I saw Sofia's head come out is indescribable and unforgettable; it is defining for me as a woman and as a mother. I hadn't been missing what I didn't know was missing, but now I understand what other women have meant for us to experience when they defend our right to have natural childbirth. They put Sofia on my chest, then whisked her off to be cleaned up and given oxygen. Her oxygenation levels were down, and she stayed in the intensive care unit for forty-eight hours. (Of course, I was convinced that they were down *because* they took her away from me.) I was vaguely surprised to find out that I'd torn and took stitches to repair a class two tear. My friend presented the placenta to me, which I acknowledged respectfully. Then I was oh so tired.

Here I might remark, mildly enough, that the importance of the much-touted perfect bonding escapes me. Of course, it is important that the infant's needs be met as fully as possible (skin-on-skin, nursing, warmth, and sleep), but right then I was very grateful for the opportunity to sleep and have someone else tend to the baby.

Twenty-four hours later, I was not ecstatic, contented, or smug. I was horrified, awestruck, and mortified by the pain, and by the fact that I had been so helpless. Sure, the doula and my girlfriend kept telling me that I was doing great, that I was strong, and that I could do it and would do it, but I knew during it all and particularly that day after that Tracey and Lorene had been my anchors, and there was no way I could have done it without them, and that was almost depressing, certainly very humbling.

A year later it looks a bit different. Now that I've got the experience—it should be possible for young women to get it somehow; I must try to impart it to my daughters—I can even conceive (pardon the pun) of taking the next quantum leap, mustering the faith, and doing it myself. Even if I don't get the chance, I know I could.

‍‌

ANNA STEWART'S BIRTH STORY

YELLOW LEAVES CLASP the sodden deck as another thunderstorm passes. I am waiting for my baby to be born. It could be today or next week. He kicks over and over in the same spot, on my right side, just under my ribs. It feels like he's about to burst through, like an eagle chick breaking his shell. He is not a quiet baby. Will he be an easy child? I am eager to meet him. I've been waiting for so long. Luna, our cat, sits nearby; my lap is no longer big enough to hold him.

Two days ago my husband, Alex, and I went for a four-mile hike. I felt strong. Lots of contractions, ten minutes apart. Today I went to the doctor: I'm four centimeters dilated and ninety percent effaced. The baby's head is engaged. Will it be today?

I call my mother. Every time she hears my voice, she thinks he's been born. She's almost as anxious as I am. I tell her to check out available flights. "He'll be here soon," I say. "This week."

I'm tired of waiting. I lie on my bed, put in a tape of ocean sounds, visualize my body opening up, unfolding. I can feel his head way down in my pelvis. I ache from the pressure. I have to pee again. Another tablespoon. I go back to the bed and lie on my other side. I breathe again. In and out. "Surrender," I tell myself, "Surrender to this process. Allow yourself to open." I can almost feel his head. He's only inches away from the air, from the earth, from my arms. I make myself another cup of raspberry leaf tea. It's supposed to strengthen the uterus. I'm tired of the taste.

I doze, dreaming of holding my baby.

Four days later, after breakfast, I realize that I can no longer sit. I call my husband to come home. I burst into tears when I hear his voice. In the shower minutes later I tell my son, "This is it, my love. We'll do this together. Gently, easily. I can't wait to meet you." Blood runs down my legs, and mucus. I lean against the wall as a contraction takes my breath away.

My contractions are two minutes apart and lasting about thirty seconds. My husband changes his clothes and calls Alice, our birth assistant. I want him close to me. I am out of the shower now and walking around the house between contractions. It's hard work, but I felt exhilarated, energized, and excited.

Alice arrives and watches me through a few contractions. I am focusing on relaxing and keeping my voice low. I'm trying to remain calm. My mind can't accept that I may have hours to go. The contractions are hard, intense, and frequent. Alice asks if I feel nauseous. "Yes," I say, though I hadn't been aware I was until she asked.

"I think you're in transition," she tells us. "We had better go to the hospital." Transition? Isn't that close to when you have to push? But I had only been laboring for an hour! It was too fast, too much. My mind was trying to tell my body to follow the childbirth schedule from my class, but my body was clearly the one in charge.

Alex drives to the hospital in a record six minutes. I cling to the back seat as he changes lanes. I can't sit down. I cry out, "I feel his head. I think he's coming." The baby was moving down the birth canal, just like he was supposed to do. Later my husband told me he thought I'd deliver in the car.

Alex stops at the emergency entrance. I calmly close the car door and try to walk into the hospital. My mind is still trying to regain control. I get about twenty feet before another contraction takes over. I lean on the pay phones in the lobby and moan loudly. Heads pop out of doorways all down the hall. A nurse pushes me into a wheelchair and rushes me to maternity.

When I give the okay, the nurse checks my cervix. I am completely dilated. She tells me to start pushing, but I'm not ready yet. Alice puts on the ocean music I was listening to at home. I keep moving. Finally I get the urge and get on the bed, lying on my side. In between pushes, I notice Alex is crying. "What is it?" He can barely speak. I kiss him. "We're about to have a baby. Our baby," he whispers. That was the moment he fell in love with our son. He hadn't seen him yet, but he knew he loved him as much as anyone can love someone.

Slowly the top of our child's head emerges. Alex can see his black hair. I can only see waves of color and light. This is the hardest part. My perineum is burning. I try to breathe through the ring of fire, repeating my mantra, "Surrender." His head emerges, and he takes his first breath. I can feel his arms and legs wriggling inside of me. Then he is born, whole and beautiful. It's a miracle. Finally I get to hold my baby in my arms. I am deliriously happy. My whole body smiles. I whisper in his open, curving ear, "Welcome, Kyle. Welcome to the world. Welcome to your family. We are so glad you've come."

It seems unfair to have to push the placenta out after all that work, but I do, even with their well-intentioned pushes on my belly. I only have eyes for my new family, so I am surprised when Alice tells me that I am losing too much blood and that I need to stop it now. She makes me look at her and tells me I have to stop the bleeding right now. I close my eyes and remember my uterus, which has held my baby so well these nine months. I visualize the bleeding stopping and my uterus finally resting. It works, and they decide not to give me Pitocin and new blood. I am reconnected now, my mind in harmony with my body, my heart in bliss with my partner and my son.

Years later I listen to the sweet breathing of my three children as they sleep. As exhausted as I am, I want to stay in that space forever, where my children are safe and warm and I can pour my love onto them through my eyes and hands and breath. I feel like I have waited my whole life for such moments. My life is bigger, busier, and more demanding than I could ever have anticipated. I am no longer waiting!

Tara Hogue Harris's birth story

"I FEEL LIKE I want to push," I remember saying as the car rounded the corner. The birth of our son Brodie didn't go quite as we expected. My due date was August eighteenth, and while I was eager to meet the child I was carrying, I wasn't feeling especially impatient as the date drew nearer. My pregnancy had gone smoothly once the first sixteen weeks of constant nausea and vomiting had passed (alleviated somewhat by medication), and despite the summer's heat, I was feeling pretty good. I hoped to avoid drugs and interventions and wanted to labor at home as long as safely possible, picturing long hours of walking or showering as labor progressed and believing that I'd be more comfortable doing that at home. To assist with that we'd hired an experienced and empathetic doula to help us.

At my checkup on August twelfth, I was two to two and a half centimeters dilated, but my doctor didn't feel that anything was going to happen very soon. She said she'd see me the following week and casually talked about when they'd want to induce me should I go much past my date. Though I really wanted to steer clear of induction, I didn't worry much about it, either, figuring that a lot could happen in a week. The night of the thirteenth, I decided to make some cookies, something I'd been planning on doing for days. By eleven o'clock, I had over a hundred cookies in front of me and was ready to head to bed. My husband was out, catching up with some friends, so he joined me a few hours later.

I was up a lot that night to go to the bathroom, almost every hour instead of the usual three or four times, but nothing seemed unusual until around six AM, when I woke to go to the bathroom again. Half awake, I tried to identify what was familiar about the slight ache in my lower back and realized it was similar to the soreness I sometimes felt before my period. "Hey, that could be a sign of early labor," I thought groggily as I made my way to the bathroom again. This trip something was different. "Okay, that's my mucus plug," I thought as I peered into the toilet bowl, sure it couldn't be anything else. Time to pull out my pregnancy books to see exactly what this meant. A quick check convinced me that it didn't necessarily mean anything. It could be the beginning of labor, but it could still be days before anything happened. Knowing I wouldn't fall back asleep, I sat down to read the paper but mostly I wandered restlessly around the house.

Alerted by my early prowling, my husband, Craig, woke around seven thirty AM to ask me what was going on. By this time I was feeling something but not what I would call contractions: an intensification of the ache in my lower back but no real pain. I updated him, and we agreed that it was too early to get excited. He began to check e-mail and get ready for work, and I decided to run a bath.

I spent the next hour soaking in the tub. At the start, the ache I was feeling wasn't like contractions; there was no start or end, so I didn't think we could time anything. By about half an hour later I felt there was a definite cycle beginning, and Craig sat down to start timing them. They were sporadic at first and pretty manageable. I still had my sense of humor and found that ducking my head under the water helped as they peaked. At around nine o'clock Craig called our doula, Suzanne, to let her know what was up, but when she wasn't in, we decided there was no hurry to reach her on her cell phone just yet.

About nine thirty, I decided that I needed to walk around as the pain from the contractions increased. Craig and I were still convinced this was either false or very early labor since it had only been about an hour and a half since the first real contraction. As I paced the living room, I started to feel scared for the first time. This was real pain, and I had only been at it such a short time. I tried to remember helpful breathing techniques from yoga, Suzanne, and our hospital class but was already feeling a bit shocked at the intensity of the pain. I thought: what if this is just false labor and it hurts this much already? I didn't think I'd be such a wimp! I stopped pacing at one point to say to Craig, "Okay, if this lasts for like twelve hours, I'm going to need drugs."

I was feeling a bit fearful and shocked at the intensity of my contractions— I was unable to talk through them any longer—and I decided we should reach Suzanne on her cell. Shortly after ten AM, Craig called her on her cell phone. In a calm voice (far too calmly, I thought; why is he so calm when it's already hurting this much!?) he told her that my contractions were now about thirty seconds long and five to ten minutes apart. She reminded us of some breathing techniques and told Craig to call back when contractions were forty-five seconds long or if we wanted her to come. (She said later that she knows something is up when it's the husband who calls. She also said that she could hear me breathing

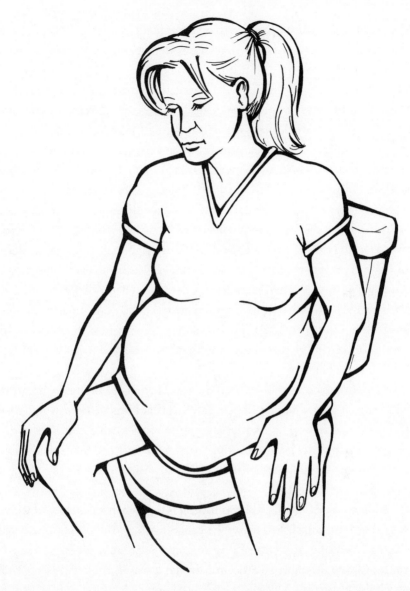

SITTING ON THE TOILET is a favorite position in labor since the toilet is the right height for the legs to be firmly supported. The lid can be left open or closed, but when it is open it allows the perineum to float freely and to bulge naturally. A pillow can be placed at the woman's back for added comfort. If the woman has begun to feel a slight urge to push, sitting in the toilet allows the baby freedom of movement to assume an optimal birthing position. Pushing in this position is very effective, too, and before moving into the actual birthing place, it is useful to do a few practice pushes on the toilet until the baby's head has crowned without slipping back in. A towel can be placed over the toilet opening if the woman is concerned about the baby falling into the water.

in the background, and she thought that I was either going to be shocked at what would come later in the labor or that things were moving very fast.)

I spent much of the next hour kneeling on the couch, my head on the armrest as I dozed between contractions. I was feeling pretty out of it but talked to Craig a bit as he continued to time things, give me sips of water, and hold my hand through contractions, still maintaining his (unnaturally, I thought) calm demeanor. I could also half hear him walking very quickly around the house as he added last-minute items to my hospital bag, and the speed of his footsteps was the only thing that told me he wasn't as calm as he seemed.

He called Suzanne again about ten thirty AM to tell her that the contractions were longer and stronger, and she confirmed that she was on her way. By about eleven o'clock, I thought I would be more comfortable sitting on the toilet, so Craig helped me into the bathroom. About eleven fifteen, I heard a distinct pop and knew that my water had broken but was too dazed to look for myself. I was also distracted by tingling in my legs and arms. Luckily, Suzanne arrived only minutes later, and after taking a quick peek calmly confirmed that not only had my water broken, there was meconium in it, so we needed to get to the hospital. When I told her about my tingling, she corrected my breathing, saying tingling was a sign of hyperventilation. Craig and I had been doing the breathing we'd learned for early labor, still not realizing that I was in the very late stages at this point, about three hours after it began. Suzanne's calm, professional presence was welcomed by both of us, since we were feeling overcome by the force of my contractions and were still unaware that things were moving far faster than usual.

An indication of how dazed I was feeling is that when Suzanne said we had to get to the hospital, I asked how we were going to get there. I couldn't imagine actually getting up and walking to a car. Suzanne decided to drive us, something she didn't normally do, but she felt it was the best way to continue to coach my breathing since she felt I was heading into transition. We left for the hospital around eleven thirty AM, Craig in the back seat with me, still calmly encouraging me.

It was about five minutes into the drive that I asked—and again I blame my foggy state on thinking this might be a good idea—if I could push. It didn't really seem related to the baby. I think I said something like I just wanted to do a sort of bowel movement push, thinking that couldn't be a bad thing. Suzanne and Craig were quite definite, though, that I should not push, and Suzanne again gave us a new breathing rhythm to help fight that urge, Craig coaching me as she drove. She called ahead to the hospital to let them know that we were coming, and they recommended that we come through the emergency entrance. Suzanne was telling us that the baby would be born before very long, but I don't remember really taking that in.

We pulled into the ambulance bay about eleven forty-five, and Suzanne escorted me as far as a wheelchair (walking was a real challenge at this point) while Craig parked her car. Since she knew where in the hospital to take me, they felt that would be best. (Craig later said he had pretty much abandoned her car since he would rather pay a ticket than miss anything. No ticket though!) Again in the elevator I asked if I could push; hey, we were at the hospital so why not, right? And again Suzanne thought I shouldn't, not in the elevator.

We were wheeled into a room, where a nurse advised me to get in the bed and get my underpants off. I heaved myself from the wheelchair and did a sort of swan dive for the bed, pulling off my underwear and shorts in one move. Craig was there by then, and we heard the good news that I was eight centimeters dilated and in full-blown transition. Suzanne kept assuring me that it was almost over, and although I liked the idea of inhaling some gas to help with the pain, things were moving too fast at that point. It felt like only a minute passed until they checked me again and found I was fully dilated, but apparently it was about ten minutes later. I was finally allowed to push!

They were monitoring the baby's heart rate by then and found that there were some decelerations, so between that and the meconium, they felt it was time to get the baby out as soon as possible. I continued to push, with Suzanne and Craig supporting me and with the assistance of the nurse. (I remember smacking her hand at one point as she took over holding one of my legs but managed to apologize a second later, and she didn't seem to hold it against me.) The doctor arrived around this time and decided that he would assist the baby out with a vacuum to speed things up. He mentioned an episiotomy, but again (and to my delight, as I didn't want one) things progressed too fast for him to do one. A few pushes later, with the help of the vacuum (and yes, that's uncomfortable, to say the least), our son was delivered. It was 12:24 PM. We had been at the hospital about thirty-five minutes.

Brodie David Hogue Harris weighed seven pounds, twelve ounces, was twenty-two and a half inches long, and despite a bit of a vacuum-induced cone head, looked perfect to us. I had experienced a bit of tearing but otherwise felt pretty good, thanks to the whirlwind labor and delivery.

Once the postbirth activity died down, the doctor and nurses had a few questions about when my labor started, when my water broke, etc. I think there was an undercurrent of irritation. They seemed to feel I had waited too long to come in because I had a doula helping me. When they heard that my water had broken only an hour before and that my first contraction was only at eight AM, the undercurrent disappeared, and we were told we'd had a precipitous labor, which apparently just means very fast. We've been told that for a second child, we'd better just park in the hospital lot at about thirty-eight weeks, or get my husband a pair of latex gloves.

LISA CLARKE'S BIRTH STORY

FIVE WEEKS OF maternity leave and still no baby. I brought work home with me, caught up on some reading, and drummed my fingers a lot. Friends said, "Enjoy the time. Sleep in." There was no way I could sleep or eat well when forty-two weeks pregnant. In fact, one afternoon my husband had to leave work and drive me around town so that I could nap in the car, the only place I was comfortable.

"Sydney Alexandra," I would say to my belly, "time to come out and play." The obstetrician had introduced us to baby-not-much-between-the-legs at our twenty-one-week ultrasound. The nursery was now filled with tiny pink dresses and butterfly walls, but our little diva was making a late curtain call.

Thursday's nonstress test at the hospital was uneventful. Even after two glasses of ice chips, Sydney didn't feel like waking up, and the contractions were minimal. The nurses proclaimed that the baby was not large and had lots of room. The ultrasound and inducement would be booked after the holiday weekend. Our midwife was calm and confident with our progress.

By Friday night I was ready to wait out the weekend. Our doula offered me a foot massage and some well-heeded advice from a mother with an eight-year-old. Also a student of homeopathic medicine, she found a remedy that might help to instigate labor. I had walked and walked, done squats, drunk raspberry leaf tea. I was willing to try anything to meet our new baby.

On Saturday at six AM, Sydney began to stir. Waking up to jarring pubic bone pain, I headed for the bathtub for a relaxing soak. By seven we called the midwife. "You've probably pulled a ligament doing those squats." But within the hour I called to my husband to start timing the pain: two to three minutes apart. This wasn't just squat!

Our midwife arrived soon after, but to my dismay I was only one centimeter dilated. She went to prepare the equipment, and our doula arrived from next door to join the home birth party. The boxes of home birthing equipment had been stored in the nursery for weeks; finally we could set up the plastic sheets and receiving blankets. We then brought the rocking chair out to the back porch so I could enjoy the May sunshine and the neighbors could enjoy my increasing moans. I rocked and rocked, trying to focus on the lessons learned in Ina May Gaskin's *Spiritual Midwifery*, but I wasn't feeling very psychedelic or high.

At one PM I started active labor. To alleviate the public bone pain, throughout the day I shifted from tub to rocking chair to slow dancing to toilet seat to shower to birthing chair. The midwife had once said to me, "A laboring woman is a lioness; we just follow her lead." Well, I was beginning to roar.

At four PM my father and stepmother joined the party. They had called en route on the highway and weren't taking "no" for an answer. When they arrived, my father called from downstairs, "Lisa, your father has arrived," just as I began vomiting into the bathroom sink. I remember my mother once saying, "When you're in labor, you don't care if you're naked in the middle of the street." She was correct.

Dinner was ordered (the smell of Chinese food was nauseating) and coffee was made, as it seemed that the night was going to be long. We tried to break the water, but the amniotic sac was very thick and wouldn't tear. After each trip to the shower or bath, someone would start brushing my hair, but I was too exhausted to be annoyed. My husband announced that a new day had begun, and I thought, "Now we'll have to get the Sunday newspaper for the time capsule."

Our doula was dozing on the bed, my husband was sprawled on the nursery floor, and the midwife waited patiently while I labored on. At three AM and at ten centimeters, I sat shivering on the toilet seat, in the only position that alleviated the pubic pain, with my head against the bathroom wall while the midwifery assistant coached me to bear down. But the contractions had stopped. The midwife offered me something to help speed up the process, then she offered me nitrous oxide, then she offered me the hospital, during the SARS outbreak. The hospital was the last place I wanted to go to. I refused everything in a haze, knowing that this baby was going to come out with sheer willpower. Later on we laughed that I was so determined but so afraid to admit that the contractions had stopped. I was convinced that if I huffed and I puffed, I would at least blow out my amniotic sac.

Finally after two hours I could feel the head with my fingers. It was amazing and incredibly motivating to know that the baby was really there. Then the real negotiations began. "But in a video I've seen a woman giving birth on the toilet," I complained. "We're not doing this in the bathroom," decreed our midwife.

My husband and doula dragged me to the bedroom, with a large head beginning to bulge out my vagina. With a few controlled pushes I shook hands with the infamous burning ring of fire. When the head came out, the midwife swiftly unwrapped the umbilical cord from the baby's neck and out she came, clean and new.

She was suctioned and rubbed to stimulate her cries, and we waited to hold her in our arms. The midwife brought her to my belly for the cord cutting, and time stopped. "Oh my," breathed my husband, "It's a boy." Laughter erupted.

Aidan Alexander was born at 5:53 in the morning as the sunrise tickled my belly. Our baby-lots-between-the-legs weighed a whopping eight pounds eleven ounces and had a full mane of chestnut hair. It was the most breathtaking and humbling moment of my life. I couldn't stop laughing, holding him in my arms.

As I tried to push out the placenta, my stepmother held Aidan in her arms. She was never able to have children of her own, and I felt honored to give this gift of life, this moment of bonding, to her. After a second threat of going to the hospital, I sat up and finally plopped the big red mess out. Time to cuddle our child and hold him to my breast.

Having a baby is truly a labor of love. Nothing could prepare me for the intensity of labor or the sacred first kiss on our child's cheek. His skin, his cry, his smell are forever ingrained in my memory.

After the birth, our midwife had to take a three-month leave of absence because her back gave out sitting on my bed for twenty-four hours. Our son has grown so quickly that at eight months of age he also put his father's back out of commission. As much as he enjoyed lounging in my belly, he is so excited and active that he never wants to sleep. With any luck, he'll walk soon and climb the magnolia tree in our backyard now being fertilized by his placenta.

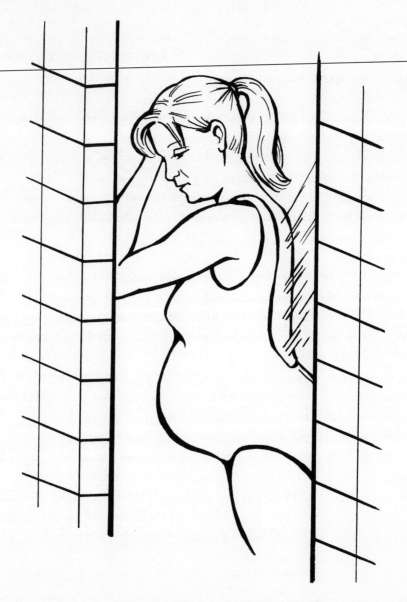

STANDING IN THE SHOWER during labor creates an optimal position for the pelvis and the cervix to open up aided by the force of gravity and the baby's head pressing on the cervix. In this position the woman has freedom of movement within her own personal space: she can sway to the rhythm of the contractions, helping ease her pain. Water, a marvelous form of pain relief on its own, can create a gentle and soothing environment for the woman to labor in, which is the key to helping her cope. The woman can direct the flow of the showerhead to any part of her body that aches. A birthing pool, where the woman can achieve full immersion in warm water, is an even more effective form of relief from the pain of the contractions since it adds weightlessness. The temperature of both the shower and the birthing pool must be kept comfortable.

Birthing Naturally Unassisted

Christina Otterstrom-Cedar

L IKE MANY MOTHERS, I have pondered birthing alone like a deer in a meadow. Could I do that and stay centered and flow with the birthing energies? Alone in the living room with my third baby giving me internal hugs, I realized that yes, I could, but I didn't want to. I wanted to share the memory of birth for it to live in more hearts than my own. So about one hour before our baby arrived, I woke up my husband. My mother heard footsteps on the floor above her and came to join us. An hour later I knelt and reached behind my legs to catch a beautiful little baby. My mother sat on the sofa in front of me. I whispered to her. "I caught my baby." She answered with reverence, "You did indeed." I had fulfilled a dream.

Years later I was told that I had an unassisted birth. This surprised me because my husband and mother were quietly present when I caught my baby.

What is the meaning of unassisted birth?

Is there such a thing? There are different definitions and perspectives on this. Technically in our society it means absence of medically trained attendants, specifically a midwife, doctor, or nurse at the birth. In the legal sense, a doula or self-educated individual does not fall under the umbrella of being medically trained.

Laura Shanley, the author of the Web site Bornfree, shares her opinion that:

> In an unassisted childbirth no one acts as midwife. Instead, the birthing woman herself determines the course of her labor. Partners or friends may participate to varying degrees, but no one instructs the woman as to how to give birth, when to push, what position to be in, etc. Occasionally suggestions may be offered, but it is assumed that the woman giving birth is the true expert on her own body.

In other cultures, unassisted birth may mean that the birthing mother is physically alone. It may also mean that she is with other people but has not been able to connect to the creative energy that is there to assist birthing women. In a spiritual sense it may mean she is separated from the greater source of life, from her personal creator, god or goddess.

My personal view is that all women are assisted, even a woman totally alone. A woman may give her sacred body, but life begets life. Sometimes the best thing we can do is disappear and let nature proceed without getting in the way. I feel that women who receive negative interference are shrouded from nature's assistance. It becomes a matter of where to put one's faith.

~ତ୍ତ~

Fear of medically unassisted birth

It is not the child who needs preparation. It is we ourselves.
—FREDERICK LEBOYER, *Birth Without Violence*

ONE OF THE MOST common assumptions people make is that having a medically unassisted birth is the most dangerous birth option available. At times this is true, but let's look more closely. Is rushing through traffic to get to a hospital safe? Are all medical procedures safe? Of course not. We delude ourselves if we think we can eliminate all risk by surrounding ourselves with technology. Birth and death are interconnected with life. There is no way to get around this fact.

In a small village, exposure to birth and death is intermingled with hearing and seeing a baby suckle the breast. It is blended with the daily experience of young and old touching hands as they gather wood for the fire. Our society tends to separate us from this open intimacy with the wheel of life. Young and old are commonly set apart in day care and old age facilities. Birth and death are largely compartmentalized and given over to the experts. Our experiential separation can leave us in the dark, feeling vulnerable. This gives fear and misunderstanding a place to grow.

Embracing the full gift of life involves coming to terms with our fears and illusions. Trudy Plaizier, a doula and childbirth educator of several years, aspires to lift the veil of mystery and fear by asking her classes, "What is your greatest fear?" A common response is "Not making it to the hospital on time." As do many midwives, Plaizier addresses this fear directly by taking time in her classes to go over what to do if a baby decides to come quickly, before medical assistance is available. Her key instructions are:

1. Find a comfortable spot to labor.
2. Create a clean space for the baby's arrival.
3. Don't travel until both the baby and placenta are delivered.
4. Don't attempt to cut the cord.
5. Let the mother hold the baby skin to skin if transportation to hospital is necessary.
6. Stay calm and recognize the beauty in the experience. If a baby is coming quickly, things are usually okay.

Staying calm is very important because fear can greatly increase the experience of pain due to the resistance created in the muscle tissue. Dr. Michel Odent writes in his book *Entering the World*, "... apart from the nature and intensity of the stimulus, the experience of pain depends on four factors: culture, anxiety, attention, and interpretation. The kind of preparation for birth we practice has an effect on all four of these factors." If a person is afraid of having a medically unassisted birth, there is all the more reason to prepare for one, to familiarize oneself and develop confidence.

During pregnancy ask your doctor or midwife to help you become familiar with palpating your baby's position. Invest in a fetoscope and get to know your baby's heartbeat; it can only bring you closer. When you are in early labor at home, it can be very reassuring to be able to monitor your baby's movements and heartbeat. Talk to your baby and describe to him or her your dream of the ideal birth. You'd be surprised at how well babies listen to their mamas. Talk to your midwife or herbologist about what tinctures to keep in the cupboard for emergencies and create a birth kit to use during labor and in the advent of birth. Find out how to use a bulb syringe or DeLee suction to clear the baby's airway. Learn different infant resuscitation techniques. Preparing for the advent of a medically unassisted birth is like having an extra life jacket in the canoe: you may never use it, but it can't hurt to bring it along.

Developing confidence helps us go beyond ourselves. We can take the nurturing steps of a mother by remembering that our baby has his or her own awareness, which can be greatly influenced by our actions and state of mind. Focusing beyond ourselves has a wide range of benefits for mother and baby. Along with the benefit of deepening the mother/infant bond, it can reduce the experience of pain. Michel Odent states that "... when the woman comes to labor without worrying about her behavior during uterine contractions and how she is controlling them, but concentrating on her baby and how she will welcome it by touch and voice, there is less risk of prolonged or painful labor due to inadequate contractions or anomalies in contraction and dilation."[1]

☙⚬

Why choose a medically unassisted birth?

WHY WOULD A woman choose to give birth without medical assistance? Often the thought comes to a person out of practicality. Not everyone has quick access to a hospital or a midwife. The thought of being in labor and traveling several hours to reach a hospital is not appealing or necessarily safe. Along with farmers and veterinarians, most people understand that transporting animals in labor can cause stress and complications. Most laboring animals do much better if they are not moved and their need for space is respected. Sometimes we forget that we, too, are animals, but most of us do well if given similar respect.

The option of leaving home days or weeks in advance of labor to be close to birthing facilities or caregiver is a choice that is challenging for some people to incorporate into their lives. The financial and emotional stress of finding appropriate accommodations and adjusting work and home life can be difficult. The option of hiring someone to travel the distance to the birth can also be beyond some people's budgets and does not guarantee that the caregiver will arrive on time.

For some people, the desire for a medically unassisted birth is not due to a lack of finances or of an available hospital or caregiver. Their practical challenge lies in trying to find a caregiver or facility to meet their needs. If a hospital or caregiver has a very high intervention rate, a mother may look at the associated risk factors and decide that she feels safer at home with people whom she trusts to respect her and her baby's needs. Incompatibility with available caregivers can make it more challenging for a mother to give herself to the birth process. Apart from any actions taken, she may feel hindered by a caregiver's inappropriate words and body language. The mother's birth option of choice may be one of "first, do no harm," putting her primary faith in the process and her secondary faith in the availability of medical facilities and personnel.

Choosing self-education and preparation for unassisted birth is not a decision people usually come to lightly or out of naïveté. Expectant birth couples have probably looked closely at all of their options. During their research on home birth, they may have slowly been filled with a sense of faith in the birth process. Over time and experiencing birth, some mothers reach a place of deep awareness of their own personal birth process. The fears that a lot of other people entertain may have been put aside. Then it is just a matter of opening up and taking another step. The choice to give birth with total privacy can bring a couple a shared experience of tender intimacy similar to the spirit in which the baby was conceived. A dad who caught his wife's baby expressed it this way: "I will never be able to describe the feeling that I experienced as I moved the baby onto my wife's stomach. We were both laughing and crying at the same time. I was so excited that I wrapped the baby up and had not even noted what sex it was. I peeked under the blanket and laughed and cried. 'We have another girl,' our second. Nothing I have ever experienced before, or shall after, will match the feeling that night."

I know that for myself, our decision to have a medically unassisted birth was first sparked because there was no midwife in the area. The idea quickly grew from there. Making the decision encouraged me to let go of relying upon others for guidance. It was easier for me to relax when I was not waiting for someone to arrive and assist me or when I was not wondering when I should leave for the hospital. I felt safer. My labors go very fast at the end and the chances of being caught alone are high. Another benefit, much milder but still of note, was that I didn't have any internal pressure to be a good patient or a good hostess; I could just be me. It is like choosing to run barefoot. You need to be aware of where to place your feet on the ground, but there are no barriers to feeling the earth. Choosing to give birth in this way brought me to a different place of awareness, openness, and intimacy with the flow of birth and creation.

I would like to clarify that "different" does not mean better. The first two births I experienced were medically supervised and deeply fulfilling, full of magic moments, great joy and growth. Every birth has its own beauty.

～∾∾～

Planning a medically unassisted birth

WHEN ONE ASPIRES to have a medically unsupervised birth, the motivation is best led by the heart, not the ego. The ego tends to be less flexible than the heart and clouds the intuition. Remember that you are not doing this alone; your baby is with you, Spirit is with you, and the lines of communication need to remain open and clear.

Unfortunately, the concept of medically unassisted births is often oversimplified as an uninformed and dangerous choice, or as a situation in which someone has been caught off guard. Planning a medically unassisted birth as your choice requires a very deep level of confidence in yourself and trust in the birth process. It is not the same for us as it was for our great-grandmothers in the pioneer days. The gifts of modern technology have a flip side. There is an extra weight of responsibility for parents due to the wide range of available choices, and there are potential legal and social ramifications of choosing a road less traveled.

Mental, emotional, and physical preparations need to have your full commitment. Proper prenatal care, including good nutrition and exercise, can prevent many birth emergencies. In a doula workshop I attended, a nurse who had worked up north said that when aboriginal women of her community became pregnant, they created a walking path. They walked upon this path daily during their pregnancy. This ritual was a key part of their prenatal care. The path symbolized their labor and birth. It was a way to honor and nurture the physical aspect of birth and connect it with the mental, emotional, and spiritual. I encourage you to explore and discover what works best for you in connecting your parts to work as a team. Perhaps it is creating a labyrinth to walk, practicing yoga, swimming, or dancing. The exploration itself can be a joy if approached with an open attitude.

Wise preparation for a medically unsupervised birth also includes you and possibly your companion becoming a student. The books *Heart & Hands* by Elizabeth Davis, *Homebirth* by Sheila Kitzinger, and *Spiritual Midwifery* by Ina May Gaskin are valuable study guides. It is also important to seek out midwives or other birthing resources that can provide excellent educational information.

Just as a person desiring a hospital birth can benefit from preparing for a surprise home birth, so can a person planning to be alone benefit from making a hospital birth plan. If you are being transported to a hospital, the last thing you need the extra stress of trying to form a spontaneous hospital birth plan.

It is crucial to be flexible and aware of potential danger signs during labor. Remember to act before a concern becomes an outright emergency. Seek validation or extra assistance. If you are lucky, you may have an arrangement in which you can phone or touch base with someone who is medically educated and receive their insight. I say "if you are lucky" because this could place your contact person in a vulnerable legal situation. You need to be fully responsible for your choices.

~·~

A safety line

Read, read, and read, yes, but you don't need a medical degree or midwifery certificate to allow your body to do what is supposed to do naturally. You don't need to go to medical school for seven years to let the waves of contractions come over your body and just be.
—RIL GILES, author, Web site <www.Unabirth.free.info>

IN MOUNTAINEERING, A climber's safety line is a piece of equipment, but when a climber is going solo, the key safety line is the ability to stay in contact with the mountain and read the climate. One of the most important safety lines of birthing is not the equipment or knowledge of emergency procedures, but knowing intuitively what is going on in your body beyond the obvious. It is being able to let go of any illusions and feel the core truth of the birthing energy. It is being able to tap into your baby's energy.

If our mind is busy on the outside, it is hard to hear the inside. For example, in one of my birth experiences, someone said, "Push." This caused an alert button to go off in my brain. I couldn't understand why someone would try to direct me unless there was danger. I had to process whether or not something was wrong. I felt pulled away from the flow of birth. I felt fear and confusion wanting to enter my sacred space. I went within and asked my inner source if everything was okay. In doing so I had to travel deeper into the earth's belly than I had ever been before. I felt peace wash over me as nature's love dissolved my being and told me everything was more than okay.

The above scenario illustrates that everyone who is with you brings along their own energy and illusions. Being aware of what those are helps you avoid being led off course. It is your choice who comes to the birth. It's important that you choose people who respect your ability to give birth. Choose people because you want them to be there rather than because they want to be there. Birth is not a place to entertain false obligations.

∾৩৶

Adaptations

MANY WOMEN FIND themselves unexpectedly having a medically unassisted birth. Some remember the experience as scary, and others remember it as wonderful. For some it was their true heart's desire, what they wanted to do all along but were afraid to openly admit or plan.

Too often it is their head's fear of judgment and condemnation that inhibits people from openly following their hearts. Sometimes nature gives them extra help to actualize their dreams. Teri Roy of Fairview, Alberta, says that although her birth didn't follow a familiar pattern, in the end "Everything worked out in exact accordance to a divine plan. I was conscious of the presence of the 'grandmothers' the whole time. Looking back, giving birth alone was really the only way I could have done it."

Sometimes nature tries her best, but we forget to take her hand. Sometimes we are yanked from her loving arms due to social circumstances. We are left aching for something we dare not embrace. A healing for one such aching mother came when she visualized giving birth to her baby all alone before she went to the hospital. While she was in labor, this birthing image gave her much needed strength and assistance. Reality can be what we embrace in our heart.

⟲⟳

Head and heart

THE QUESTIONS ARISE: How do we balance the head with the heart? How do we maintain and develop a flexible attitude within the structure of social expectations? How do we stay open and adapt our plans to the flow of birth? Everyone will have their own answers, which need to be honored. It doesn't matter whether someone else's shoe doesn't fit you. What matters is finding a shoe that fits your foot, one that will take you where you want to go, one that you can adjust or discard as you walk your path exploring, your story.

In the personal stories that follow, it is the portrayal of the power of birth that touches my inner being. Birth has its own agenda, separate from our plans. It is a power moving through us. Being open and aware of the flow of birth is like traveling the path of a river. If the river is deep and wide with whirlpools, you might choose to be in a boat with a crew helping you row. However, if the river is steady and clear with a sandy bottom, you might choose to float naked and unencumbered, while keeping alert to changes in the current. It's also important to remember that just as currents can change, being in a boat doesn't mean you are safe. Boats can tip. The energy of a river is to be respected.

There are many similarities in how different rivers and different births flow, but each river, each birth, is unique and follows its own course. Each river, each birth is a sacred part of life, and I give thanks to those who have shared their stories in this book for they help to weave a beautiful web.

Fifth blessing

I felt a strong internal hug fade away
Soon, Sweet Baby, Soon
I half ran down the hill
Then stopped
And dropped to my knees
In the thicket, by the river
My mother, the Earth
Surged through me
As I gripped
Her pale Green hair
The fresh, raw smell of nature
Enveloped my senses
I sang a welcome
To the miracle within my womb.
Turning, I leaned back into my lover's body
Encircling my vulva with my hands
I melted . . .
Into the Earth's deep void.
I sank below.
My body was not my own, it had linked with
The Earth's energy
We were one.
A fire rushed through us
We Yowled
A flash flood followed.
We bellowed.
Oh Glorious release!
Then a voice sliced through
The earth's crust,
A shovel in Paradise,
Separating me, from her.
I sought solace by diving down
deeper
deeper

down
Into the earth's belly bowl
PEACE greeted me.
The earth's love dissolved
My being
Life burst forth
From darkness into light
At the end of a bellow
So be it.

CHRISTINA OTTERSTROM-CEDAR is the author of the booklet *Outside Wombs*. Her mothering journey began in 1984 with the conception and loss of twins at five months' gestational age. She has given birth to four more children, two of whom were born at home without medical assistance. She has a physical education degree and a fine arts diploma, and her experiences include being a doula, a La Leche League leader for sixteen years, a communications skills instructor, a social services case worker for abused children, a storyteller, a wildlife guide, an artist, and a facilitator for personal growth workshops.

∽

MARLENE WAECHTER'S BIRTH STORY

THIS IS THE story of Rachel's birth. The first clue that I was pregnant again was sore nipples and breasts. I was puzzled because I had not had any problems so far nursing Becky, either when she was born or over the past eighteen months. I could not figure out why my breasts would be hurting this far into the nursing relationship. I mentioned this to my obstetrician one day when I was working at his office. (I taught home birth education classes there.) He asked if I had done a pregnancy test. I answered, "No." I had been faithfully checking my cervical mucus and had not had any signs of fertile mucus, which I knew usually preceded one's first menstrual period after a birth, let alone a period itself. I had also been charting my basal temperature and had not seen any patterns that looked like the return of fertility, so the possibility of pregnancy had not even crossed my mind.

Sure enough, I was pregnant. Since I had not had any periods yet, we could not set my due date that way but only by the size of my uterus. This was 1978 and sonograms were around but were not routine, plus we did not have insurance, so we never did have one.

We figured that I would have the baby sometime in February or March or maybe even at the beginning of April, if you give a two-week window on either side of the due date, whenever that was. My labor with Becky had been seventy very intense minutes, from the first sign of labor with my water breaking until she was out, breathing and peeing. Since I lived way out in the country and did a lot of driving, I thought I had two choices: either hole up at home for possibly three months or be prepared to have this baby anytime and anywhere. I chose the latter. By the end of January, I had covered my mattress with plastic and had disposable pads, gauze pads, towels, washcloths, baby blankets, along with a cord bander, hemostats, and scissors together in a bowl for the placenta, all inside a trash bag that went everywhere with me. I was prepared!

Around Christmas I started having Braxton Hicks contractions, especially when I was with someone else in labor. Sympathy contractions, I called them.

I was in the habit of attending monthly staff meetings at the obstetrician's office, which was over an hour from my house. At the January meeting, one of the midwives suggested that the next meeting be at my house. Everyone agreed.

On February nineteenth, I was having so many contractions that I made my husband stay home from work, but they never developed into real labor contractions. We even took a long walk after dinner, but no luck. The next morning was the day of the staff meeting at my house and it began like all the others. Becky woke about six AM; I changed her diaper and tucked her into bed next to me. She nursed, and we both fell back to sleep for a few more hours as my husband and son got up, got themselves breakfast, and went off to work and school respectively. Before he left, my husband asked me if I thought he should stay home again, but I told him no. I had not had any contractions at all since falling asleep the night before, so he might as well go. Then back to sleep I drifted.

I was rudely awakened by a strong contraction. I opened one eye. It was eight-forty AM. I quickly closed my eye and promptly fell back to sleep. Whoa! Another contraction woke me again. I peeked at the clock: nine o'clock. "Only one and a half hours before the meeting. I better get up and dressed and clean up the house," I told myself. The spirit was willing, but the flesh was weak. Back to sleep I fell. A third time a contraction woke me at nine-twenty AM, and I thought to myself, "Hmmm, pretty strong, but twenty minutes apart. At this rate I will not have the baby until tomorrow. My contractions with Becky were two minutes apart. This one will take ten times as long!" In the meantime, I had to get ready for a meeting. But Becky was nursing again, so I thought I would just lie there until she finished. Once again, I promptly fell back to sleep.

Next thing I knew, it was nine forty AM, and this time, instead of a contraction waking me, nature was calling me to the bathroom. I slid a finger down the side of my breast into Becky's mouth to gently break the suction, then quietly slid out of bed, trying not to wake Becky, and rushed to the bathroom just in time to empty my bladder and bowels. I had a very crampy diarrhea that kept coming and coming, so I called my husband to turn around and come home. Still not realizing this was it, I thought I had food poisoning or a stomach virus or something. I just knew that I was miserable.

I was finally fully awake and realized how close I was cutting it for the meeting. Becky awoke and was not happy that I had abandoned her before she was ready to stop nursing. I sat her down in front of a bowl of cereal, called my friend and neighbor, Kate, and asked her to come and help me take care of Becky and vacuum the living room before the doctor and the rest of the midwives showed up for the meeting. Then I rushed back to the toilet, grabbing my clothes as I went. I sat on the toilet, got dressed, and brushed my teeth from there as I was still having diarrhea.

It was ten AM. Finally a pause in the action. I wiped and saw a bloody show. "Hmmm," I thought, "Has this diarrhea dilated me any?" I checked: no cervix; none at all. I was complete. Diarrhea or no, I was not having this baby on the toilet. I waddled into bed. Then I remembered the supplies, which were in the bedroom but not within reach. I just could not get back up to get them. Dealing with contractions was taking everything I had. I prayed, "Dear Lord, send someone to walk through that door to help me!" With that there was a knock. I could not get up so I screamed, "Come in, whoever you are!" It was Kate and her three-year-old, Mikey. She started to take off his coat, mittens, and boots. I screamed again, "Come here!"

She walked into the bedroom, saw about a three- to four-inch circle of head showing at my bottom, and said, "Oh my God. What do I do?" I was breathing so hard I could not answer, so I started pointing to my bags in the corner. Like a game of charades, she grabbed at things, "Is it this? Is it this?" with me shaking my head no, until she hit the right pile! She got a pad under me just before the rest of the head came out. Then I blurted out as much information as I could between contractions.

In the meantime, Mikey had disrupted Becky from her cereal, and they were running around the house. They were running through our bedroom as the head was crowning. I had prepared Becky for the birth by showing her pictures of a baby being born, so when she saw it, she came to a screeching halt at my bottom. Mikey, not having the preparation Becky had, had no idea what was happening and wanted to keep playing tag. He said, "Come on, Becky!" Becky replied, with wisdom far beyond her two years, "No. Baby—BABY!" So Mikey stopped and watched too.

Kate caught the baby on the very next contraction at ten minutes after ten. At ten twenty, one of the midwives showed up and right behind her was my husband. He was crestfallen to find Rachel born and nursing already. Promptly at ten thirty, the rest of the midwives, who had carpooled, showed up right on time for the meeting. The obstetrician was busy on a hospital delivery and never made it out of town. We finally got the placenta delivered and the cord cut and proceeded with the meeting. Not much business got discussed that day, but it was a meeting we will never forget. Rachel weighed in at nine pounds, eleven ounces. I had no tears, either! And this was the "tiny, preemie baby" my nutritionist warned me I would have if I ignored her advice to wean Becky. The day after the birth I went to the health department to file the birth certificate and just had to stop by the nutritionist's office to show her off!

⟡

Christy Kramer's birth story

I FELT LIKE a failure over the caesarean section. I was induced with Pitocin for no reason other than the physician's convenience. When I had pushed for only an hour, the physician decided that I had cephalopelvic disproportion (CPD)— the baby is too big to fit through the mother's pelvis—and told me that I needed a caesarean section. Being young and naïve, I agreed without getting all the information about the risks, necessity, and so on.

Later when I found out I was pregnant with my son, I knew I wanted to try to have a vaginal birth. I called around to various physicians, but no one would accept me as a patient because having a vaginal birth after a caesarean was "dangerous." So I tried local birth centers, but they would not accept me, either, for the same reason. Then a friend told me about home births and encouraged me to find a midwife who would help me have the birth I desired. So I did research for weeks, talked to midwives and to gain encouragement, information and support, talked to other women who had had vaginal births after caesareans. The more I read the more excited I became.

Unfortunately in the state where I live, lay midwives are banned from practicing home births, but after a little digging, I found a woman named Karen who was willing to help me. She seemed to have a spark about her when we spoke on the phone, and I trusted her with ease. We met for an interview a couple of weeks later, and after our initial visit I knew she was the one to help me have my home birth. Unfortunately, she lived two hours away, but she assured me that there would probably be plenty of time for her to get there.

Although the pregnancy was progressing smoothly, my husband, Jay, was a little hesitant to fully accept the idea of home birth. I agreed to keep seeing the obstetrician who I had had with my daughter so my husband would feel more comfortable. I did not tell my obstetrician of my plans to birth with a midwife at home. I did tell her that I wanted a vaginal birth after caesarean, to which she replied, "You could not even give birth to a six-pound baby. What makes you think you can give birth this time?" I was hurt and angry over the statement, but it just encouraged me even more to deliver at home. She told me that surely my uterus would rupture and discouraged me from even trying.

Nevertheless, I continued to see her for monthly appointments, but they were short and to the point. I did not bring up the subject of vaginal birth after caesarean again.

My visits with my midwife were so much different from my visits with the obstetrician. My midwife was personal and friendly, asking how things were going with my life. Often we met at her home or mine. My obstetrician would see me for about ten minutes, but my visits with the midwife would last for at least an hour. Karen never did anything that I did not feel comfortable doing. I enjoyed this about her and felt that we actually had a developing friendship instead of the hostile relationship I had with my obstetrician.

As I approached the thirty-fourth week of pregnancy, I went in for another visit with my obstetrician. While doing my routine weight and blood pressure check, the nurse asked me if I had scheduled my caesarean section yet. I was confused and reminded her that I had told them in the beginning that I wanted a vaginal birth. Then she told me that the hospital does not allow vaginal births after caesareans. I told her that I had spoken to them about seven months ago and understood that they did allow them. She was not sure if the rule had perhaps changed, so she said she would ask the physician about it. I was dumbfounded. I knew that they were talking about it, but I did not think I would have to face it. I never thought that I would not be given a choice of how to birth.

When my physician came in and did the routine examination, I brought up the issue of vaginal birth after caesarean. She said that the hospital will allow them but it had to be natural: with no drugs. That was fine with me, not that it mattered at that point, because I had already decided to deliver at home anyway. Then she said that we would do an ultrasound that week to see how much the baby weighed. She said that if he was over six pounds, ten ounces (my daughter's birth weight), she thought it would be "foolhardy" to do a vaginal birth. I did not say much, but I thought she was full of crap. She made it very clear that I was not capable of birthing a baby vaginally.

That is when I made the decision. I was tired of lying. I was tired of her negativity, and I did not need that going into a home birth. So I decided to leave her practice completely and arrange total care with my midwife. I cancelled my ultrasound appointment, obtained my medical records from the office, and wrote my physician a letter, telling her that the care I received from her was not what I was looking for and that I had decided to deliver at home with a midwife. I sent the letter off on Friday, September fifth.

The weekend continued normally, and on Sunday we went to dinner with my mother. I was feeling tired and irritable and was having light contractions all day. I was used to it because I had been having them off and on for about a week. We made it through dinner and went home to relax. As nightfall came, Jay and I decided that it had been a while since we made love, and we wanted to be together at least one more time before the baby came. Little did we know how right we were.

Around ten PM, I had taken a first dose of evening primrose oil as Karen had suggested to help tone my uterus. Skylar was getting tired, so I lay down with her to nurse her to sleep. As I did, I noticed that the contractions were becoming stronger and more frequent. They still were not lasting very long, but I was becoming a bit concerned. I looked outside and commented to Jay that I wondered if the full moon had anything to do with my contractions. I had heard that some women are sensitive to weather changes and thought maybe I could be one of them.

As Skylar drifted off to sleep, I was starting to breathe through the contractions, but I still was not sure if I should be worried about them. Suddenly at about eleven o'clock, I felt a strong contraction followed by a pop in my abdomen and intense pain. That is when I thought something could really be happening. I knew that many women describe the feeling of their water breaking as a popping sensation. I did not feel any leaking, so I went to the bathroom to check. I had to pee anyway, but I noticed that before I even tried to pee, I was already leaking a small stream of clear fluid. I knew then that it was my water.

I called Karen and told her the situation. I was still unsure about it. I thought perhaps I had just a small leak in my amniotic sac and that it was nothing to be too concerned about. I explained that it was just a small leak and that my contractions were still only about ten to twenty seconds long. She seemed suspicious and said she was going to call the other midwife and call me back. About ten minutes later, she called back and told me she was going to come down. I told her I was glad because as I was talking to her, out gushed the rest of my amniotic fluid.

By just after midnight Monday morning, Karen was on the road and kept in touch with us on our progress. Since my water had broken, my labor had gone from zero to ten in a matter of minutes. The contractions were now lasting about thirty to forty seconds and were only about two minutes apart. I decided to sit in the tub, but it did not seem to help much. However, when I faced a few contractions on land, the tub seemed like the lesser of two evils.

I was in intense pain, and just when I thought it could not get worse, it did. I started to have doubts about my ability to handle the pain. My rational mind fought with me, saying that maybe I was in transition. It is common for women to start having doubts during that period of labor. The midwife was not there yet, so I had no way of checking to find out. I just had to keep going. After a few more contractions, I was in extreme pain and told Jay that I could not do it anymore. I did not want to go to the hospital, but I could not deal with the pain. Jay told me, though, that he was not going to take me to the hospital. He said that if I did go, I would just regret it. He reminded me of why I was doing this home birth and said that I was doing great.

Shortly before one AM, I noticed that my contractions were ending with pressure on my rectum. I knew this could signal the pushing phase, but I did not say anything to Jay about it because I was not sure. I wished Karen were there so she could check me. I decided I would do better if I got out of the tub because it was not helping much anymore.

As soon as I stepped out of the tub, I was overcome with pain and dropped to my knees beside the bed. I had labored on my hands and knees in sort of a frog position when I was in the tub and thought it would be the best position on land too. As soon as I got down on my knees, I hunched over the bed and let out an unearthly primal scream. I felt the overwhelming urge to push like I had always heard about. I had not experienced it with my first labor, but this time there was no doubt about what I was feeling. I left my normally serene and calm body and instantly was transformed into a primitive banshee with each contraction. I felt like I was in a different world now. I had no control over my body anymore. It was only what it was and not what I wanted it to be. I was not who I had imagined I would be. My contractions came one on top of the other without rest, and with each one I screamed as loudly as I could. I did not care who heard me.

After about thirty minutes of pushing, I could feel the baby progressing down the birth canal. Jay was on the phone with Karen, who still was about fifteen minutes away. Unfortunately, at that point my screaming woke Skylar up, and Jay went to go comfort her and try to get her back to sleep. I remained in the bedroom for those few minutes, still pushing. Only this time, with each push I felt that burning sensation that I had heard about, and I knew Elijah would be here soon. Each time I felt a sting and would feel his head start to inch out but then slip back in.

For a second I thought maybe I would not be able to push him out. Maybe my physician was right. Maybe I was just too small and I would never be able to give birth vaginally. But during that second, my rational mind broke in again and told me that I could do it. I had made it this far, and I was going to get the chance to fulfill my dream. That baby was ready to come, and I would push him out. With the next contraction I pushed with all my might, and I felt another popping sensation. I knew his head had come out.

I yelled for Jay to come in because I knew I could not deliver him myself while I was on my hands and knees. He had put the television on for Skylar to keep her calm and was on the phone with Karen. She was pulling into our neighborhood as they spoke. He came into the bedroom and exclaimed out loud, "Oh my God, his head it out!" I said, "I know! That's why I called you!" In the next moment I pushed again with all my might, screaming into my bed. Jay was still on the phone with Karen, but he put the phone down and reached around the baby's head and gave a small tug. I felt another pop, his slippery body released from mine, and I knew it was over. He fell into his Daddy's arms and gave a startled cry. Jay wrapped him up in a blanket, set him on the bed, and hung up the phone. He left for a moment to open the front door, where Karen was waiting. Just as she came into our driveway, she heard the baby's cry over the phone.

I rolled over onto my back, and Karen came in to greet us. I lay there sobbing over my new miracle. Karen gave me a hug and laid my son on my chest. I made a joke about what good timing she had, and we laughed. He was perfect, although he looked so small. I had forgotten just how small newborns are.

Jay was relieved to have Karen there to take over and let us rest. She checked the baby over. About six minutes after he was born, I delivered the placenta with ease. Everything was intact, including the membranes. Elijah and I both looked good, although my bed looked like I had delivered in the middle of the Red Sea. Elijah measured nineteen inches long, and he weighed seven pounds, two ounces. He was born at thirty-five and a half weeks, but I think that the dates may have been wrong.

Despite all the pain, it was worth it. I lived my dream: I delivered my son the way I wanted to, the way that I was supposed to. I proved the physician and the naysayers wrong. While it was not my intention, it was a triumph. It was an empowering, inspirational, simply miraculous experience that I will never forget. I watched God answer my prayers right before my eyes, and I will be forever grateful for it.

Incidentally, Monday afternoon I received a call from the physician's office asking me to verify my leaving the practice. I confirmed it and said that I did not feel comfortable with her care and her choices for my labor and delivery. She asked me who the midwife was that I was going with, and I declined to answer. (I did not want Karen to get in trouble for practicing medicine without a license.) She wished me a curt, "Good luck with your delivery." I said, "Actually, he was born last night." She seemed a bit miffed as I explained that I had had a vaginal delivery and that my husband had caught our son. She gave me a halfhearted congratulations and hung up the phone as I giggled about the conversation.

LANNA PALSSON'S BIRTH STORY

TAIT'S LIFE BEGAN in Venice, Italy. He shared the news with his mother sixteen days later by appearing as the second blue mark on the stick.

Over the days following this discovery, my love and protective instincts toward this new life I'd been chosen to bring into the world grew exponentially. I wanted to have the healthiest pregnancy possible. I immediately said good-bye to the second cup of coffee, skipping coffee altogether on days I wasn't craving it. My diet was already healthy, but I read everything about vegetarian pregnancy that I found, making improvements if needed. Gone, too, was the glass of red wine I so enjoyed with dinner. Overnight I was transformed from the quintessential adventurous, free-spirited single woman—kayaking solo in northwestern Ontario, sailing on a tall ship in the north Atlantic, or whatever my heart led me to do—to becoming somebody's mother, with all the associated responsibilities that go with the title.

Somebody's mother, somebody's mother. Regardless of how often I repeated it, somehow it still sounded foreign to me. I would have to go to a hospital, in my opinion a filthy cesspool of disease. After being involved in a motor vehicle accident in 1998, I was all too familiar with the health care system. There had to be a better solution. I decided on a midwife.

I wanted a home birth, believing that the mainstream medical model would not be imposed upon me here. I met the midwife, and we discussed my situation. She assured me that the hospital had beautiful newly renovated birthing suites, and since my social support network was limited, I got the feeling that she preferred I go there. According to her, using one of the birthing suites meant that I would feel like I was at home yet have the safety measures of a hospital just in case. Initially I agreed. I felt in no position to be disagreeable. After all, I wanted her to like me since she'd be "delivering" my baby. Something didn't feel right though.

From early on I read everything I could about pregnancy and birth. My heart wanted to do this right, and my head was telling me that most of what I was reading that seemed culturally normal was wrong. There were two books that stood out as different: *Birth Without Violence* by Frederick Leboyer and *Gentle*

Birth Choices by Barbara Harper. I needed to learn more. I realized that this wasn't all about avoiding the hospital. The new life growing in me deserved the best possible start in life. I felt hypocritical eating healthy and exercising in order to have a healthy pregnancy so that I had the best chance of a healthy baby and successful recovery, but it mattered how this new soul arrived into the world. There was more to it than both of us simply being healthy.

I had lots to think about, and I needed to be straight with my midwife. I didn't want to offend her, since I felt that I should feel lucky even to have one. I had heard that many women weren't able to get a midwife and received their prenatal care through an obstetrician. I talked to the midwife, explaining that I truly wanted a home birth and that I had some issues with hospital settings. She informed me that the local regional health authority regulated midwives and required two to be present during home births. She would ask around and let me know.

I wanted a labor tub to use during labor. I had read that it eased the perception of contractions. I had also read that some people gave birth in the water. I wasn't too sure about that; I'd have to learn more.

Late July I attended my first childbirth class. It was run by a doula group. I was certain that I'd be surrounded by like-minded parents. But I was the only one who knew what a doula was, and these women were just weeks away from their due dates. How could they get this far along and not know what a doula was? I was the only person who wanted a home birth, the only one dead set against drugs. They listened to my birth day wishes with that deer-in-the-headlights look of awe and disbelief. I felt like a freak.

So far I had read about twenty-five books. The ones that had some impact during these weeks were *Prenatal Parenting* by Frederick Wirth, MD, and *The Secret Life of the Unborn Child* by Thomas Verny, MD, and John Kelly.

My next appointment with my midwife was approaching. I felt optimistic that I'd get the answer I wanted. No such luck. It was summer, and people were on vacation; she wasn't able to give me an answer at that time. In September she still hadn't asked around. There was a meeting the next day with all the midwives, and she would get an answer. Everything was fine as best she could tell—I had declined all prenatal testing—and she told me I was a boring pregnant person. This was a compliment. All my belly measurements were on track, I was gaining weight well, and my blood pressure was excellent. I was as low risk as possible.

The night of my first prenatal yoga class, I was eager to meet other moms-to-be. At the end of class some of us were talking. I mentioned that I wanted to find a childbirth class and shared my previous experience, hoping to find a referral where I might meet similarly motivated people. The yoga instructor said that a class had just started. I'd missed one class, but I'd read so much that she felt I could join late.

The next night I went. I was very impressed. Finally I'd met women who weren't in line for an epidural. I was relieved. I didn't feel like an alien. There were videos available to watch at home. I picked one about home birth since I planned on having one. I was also able to get a copy of Ina May Gaskin's *Spiritual Midwifery*, a book I'd seen referred to in other books but until now had not been able to find. I was starting to feel well-informed about my choices surrounding childbirth, and sensed that I was correct in my initial feelings that mainstream medicine is doing it all wrong. I was starting to realize that I was definitely intent on avoiding the hospital. I felt this was the best way to protect my baby from somebody's potential error, mistake, or intervention, which seemed far more likely to occur in a hospital than at home.

I came across a Web site for the Association for Safe Alternatives in Childbirth (ASAC). Dr. Odent was coming to Edmonton—next week. I called ASAC hoping that there would be space for one more. A trip wasn't in my budget, but this baby deserved to have a well-informed mother. My lucky day: ASAC had space, the airline had seats, and—wow—the woman I spoke to at ASAC said I could spend the night at her place.

Dr. Odent's views on women and childbirth made sense. He explained that the needs of a woman in labor are basic and simple: do not stimulate her neocortex. To accomplish this he advised respecting four things: converse minimally, keep the lights low, reduce the number of observers, and avoid raising her adrenaline. These sounded obvious to me, and I realized sadly that this is exactly the opposite of what most women experience. Odent also spoke about the uterus and its ability to do all the work to birth a baby if it is allowed to do so. No pushing is required. Essentially it will expel its passenger when the time is right. This trip raised my confidence level and helped me trust that I intuitively knew how to birth.

Thirty-three weeks, thirty-two centimeters of belly, and blood pressure dandy. There was no answer regarding the home birth; I don't recall the reason.

I was excited. November was just around the corner; this could be my last whole month of being pregnant.

At thirty-five weeks, the midwife asked if I'd taken the tour. I said, "No, I wasn't planning to go to hospital." She thought it important to be familiar with the hospital just in case. I agreed to take the tour. We met there the next week. During the tour, I commented on how dirty the floors were; she assured me that they would be clean when I went into labor. I also noticed that the lovely, homelike birthing suites she had mentioned were nothing of the sort. They were hospital rooms with hospital equipment hidden behind wood veneer fixtures. As for the labor tubs, they weren't in the individual rooms as I was led to believe; they were in another room with more wood veneer. To use the tub, I would have to get dressed to go back to my room or strut through the hallways naked. So much for a woman's need for privacy during labor. At this point, the midwife told me that she just couldn't find a second midwife so I couldn't have my home birth. I was angry. I insisted on a home birth.

I was not impressed with the turn of events, and a meeting was scheduled between the midwife, the regional health authority, and me. They had rules and no intention of bending them. Decisions were made based on established guidelines. Common sense was not permitted. I was asked point blank whether I intended to pursue home birth. I told them I did. I was extremely healthy and saw no reason why I couldn't.

The midwife pronounced me "discharged from care." Pardon me?! "We have no choice. The regional health authority and the midwifery legislation permit midwives to practice and require that they limit their practice to low risk clients." Wait a minute. Wasn't I as low risk as possible? No, I was now labeled high risk, and therefore they had to transfer my care to an obstetrician. What had changed to elevate my status to high risk? "Attitude." According to them, my insistence on home birth jeopardized the life of both my child and myself. Unless I agreed to the hospital, I would have to continue my care elsewhere. I appeased them and agreed to the hospital (despite having no intention of keeping my agreement); doing so allowed me to keep the midwife.

It was agreed that I would be "permitted" to labor at home and transfer to the hospital for delivery. I was annoyed at how this was unfolding, but decided to let it go. I had confidence in my ability to birth at home but acknowledged that if the unexpected occurred and I was required to go to the hospital, it would be nice to see a familiar face. My baby was due in two and a half weeks. There was no benefit to getting stressed over this losing battle.

The appointment wasn't over. Since I had "wisely decided" that hospital birth was the best choice for the health and safety of my baby, I was still a client and entitled to a prenatal checkup. Thirty-seven weeks and thirty-one centimeters—"Oh, this isn't good." She also estimated that I would continue past my due date by about ten days. I knew perfectly well that everything was fine. It was a different person measuring, one that had an interest in me needing her services. What better way to reinforce this than by finding a problem. I declined the offer to have a fetal assessment. I had no interest in bombarding my baby with ultrasound waves.

I had just days left, and I was basically prepared. I had the car seat and all the assorted paraphernalia for a newborn. The labor tub was rented, and I'd reviewed lists of things recommended for home birth in various books. On November seventeenth, I called a woman in Saskatchewan to obtain a copy of Laura Kaplan Shanley's book *Unassisted Childbirth*. I explained my situation and that I was due next Tuesday, and we shared a good laugh. I got the book two days later. One passage was of particular significance to me. I recall feeling strong, powerful, and confident when I read the following excerpt:

> Autonomy means independence. The term is generally used by social scientists, theologians or psychiatrists to refer to the individuated, self-actualized or authentic human being, a self-governing and self-defining person subject primarily to his own laws of being and deeply sensed goals and values. This does not mean that autonomous individuals reject social customs out of hand but rather that their locus of control, their reference point for decision making rests within ... autonomous persons consciously author their own lives.
> —MARSHA SINETAR, "Living Happily Ever After"

On Friday the twenty-first, I met with the doulas, S. and J., who would be attending my birth. With the recent twist of events, there were things we needed to discuss. They were wonderful to agree to attend my birth, especially since the midwives wouldn't. Though I know that I could have done it solo, it was reassuring to know that they supported me and were willing to help me if required. My needs were simple; I did not intend for this to be a complicated event. We reviewed likes and dislikes and laughed when we agreed that telling someone to relax had the opposite effect. I explained that my plan was to labor in my tub with lots of candles. I had purchased a CD titled *Music to be Born By* and wanted that playing. I explained that I wanted to be left alone and would

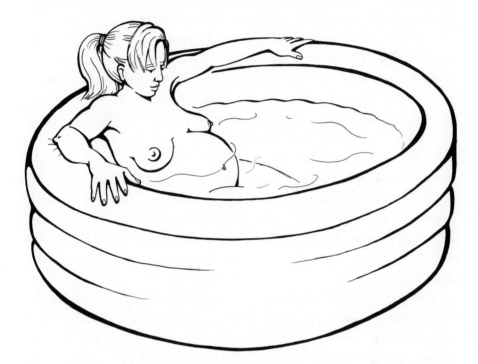

BIRTHING POOLS can be a great aid for pain relief and freedom of movement during labor. Floating in the pool, her pregnant weight lifted by the water, the woman moves unencumbered by the force of gravity or by social inhibitions. Within the confines of the pool she has a sense of being in her own private world and begins to behave by instinct, assuming any position that she feels is optimal for her and her baby. Depending on the woman, immersion in warm water can have a significant reduction in the amount of pain experienced in labor, and since it helps her relax, it also helps the release of endorphins, which are the body's natural painkillers. The mechanics of the birth are aided by having the body suspended in water, preventing perineal tears and giving the baby a gentle transfer from amniotic water into water again. The more relaxed a woman is during labor, the better equipped she is to handle the pain of contractions. She can be in the pool during active labor only, or she can stay and give birth in it. It is safe for a baby to be born in the water once it is brought immediately but gently to the surface. Babies are born without their lungs expanded because they are surrounded by amniotic fluid for nine months, getting their oxygen through the umbilical cord. It is only when they hit the cold air outside the pool that their breathing reflex is stimulated.

call them into the room if needed. The details were worked out. They were attending a workshop that weekend and S. had a talk with my baby, speaking up close to my bare belly—the Starbucks patrons were no doubt surprised!—explaining they were excited to meet but that this was a busy weekend. She explained times that would be convenient. We could only hope that this baby knew how to tell time.

Saturday was laundry day, loads of flannel blankets and tiny clothes. Sunday I went to the art gallery and then to a friend's house for dinner and a movie. I left for home around ten PM. I had a couple of contractions on the way home; they weren't a big deal. At home they continued. I'd heard that lots of women have Braxton Hicks contractions, so I thought I'd wait to see how these progressed. I lit a few candles and kept myself busy.

By two AM, I suspected this was it. The contractions weren't letting up, and were getting stronger. I hopped in my tub. This was the reason I'd rented it! I'd heard that singing in labor helped the progression; I can't sing, so I hummed. The only song I could think of was *Silent Night*. I didn't want to bother the doulas yet. At about three thirty AM, I wanted more water. When I stood up I realized (and appreciated) how much the water was taking the edge off the contractions.

I think the remainder of my experience could be defined as "freight train" labor. If the doulas were coming, now was the time. I called at three forty-five AM. There was no answer, so I left a message. A few minutes later my phone rang. I guess she could tell by my voice how I was doing. She said she was on her way and hung up.

Now that I'd called the doulas, the next obstacle was: how were they going to get into the building? I felt in no shape to make it down three flights of stairs and unlock the door to the building. I was comfortable with having the baby alone, but I wanted the companionship of the doulas. My friend R. had a spare key to my apartment, so I called him. I explained the situation; he headed over right away arriving, around four twenty AM. He turned on every light. He was tense because the doulas hadn't yet arrived. I sent him downstairs to wait. I hoped he could relax. I didn't want to divert my focus to reassure him.

Around five AM, I heard the doulas J. and S. arrive. J. asked if she could get me anything. "Light. Off." The hallway light was mercifully eliminated. They replaced candles that had burned out. I was in my groove. They brought me the ice cubes of red raspberry tea that I had prepared.

I was well on my way into "laborland," and as vivid as some things are, others are vague. I know that they reminded me to pee and helped me to the toilet. Since I didn't know when to push, I didn't. I understood that when the right time came, the urge would be undeniable. I'd read that pushing early could cause the cervix to swell and result in complications. I trusted that my body knew how to give birth. Contractions were intense but tolerable. I assumed that they would become more intense at some point. I continued to let myself go and flow with the contractions. I used a deep, low moan to get through the contractions, and it worked. I think I beckoned for J. and S. to keep me company and hold my hand at this point. I remember that they told me I was beautiful and that my uterus was working amazingly effectively and efficiently to push my baby out. I could feel my baby making its way out; I felt like I was being split in two halves.

Suddenly the water was too hot for me, and S. added pails of cold water to the tub. It felt like baby was almost out. I guess I was having a water birth since I had no intention of getting out of the tub at that point. My only minor regret is that I didn't reach down to feel the baby's head emerging. I recall feeling hot, so I kept my arms out of the tub, hanging over the edge to keep cool; I didn't want to get them wet with hot water, which makes no sense now. The water was actually on the cool side, thanks to S.

Suddenly I was in the midst of the most uncontrollable urge to get this baby out. It hurt, but I didn't care; I was pushing. I couldn't believe my baby was almost here. I reached to feel if the cord was around the baby's neck. There was no cord. I gave another push, and baby was here. I brought the baby up from beneath the water, so tiny, so perfect, eyes open wide and gazing. A huge yawn, brief smile, and a short bleating howl.

We snuggled close; J. and S. got a blanket. We had done it! This baby knew how to be born; I knew how to give birth. I glanced at the clock. It was 7:41 AM.

At 7:43, in walked R.; he'd gone for breakfast. He got my camera and took a couple of photos. The flash bothered the baby, so we didn't take any more. After twenty minutes or more I still hadn't checked to see whether we should be saying he or she. It's a he! My beautiful baby boy—he was perfect. We got some help getting out of the tub, curled up together in some warmed blankets, and J. brought a fruit smoothie. I needed this nourishment. S. got some arnica for me. They took great care of us. I'd asked them to call R. just before the baby arrived. If it hadn't been for him having a key to the building, I'd have called all of them myself, after the baby arrived.

I called the midwives to cancel the next day's appointment, which was my due date. When one of the midwives returned my call, she asked what was wrong. I said nothing was wrong, that I wouldn't need the appointment, that he was here and he was beautiful. This took a moment to sink in. She said, "What do you mean?" and I said, "He was born this morning!" I explained that labor was easy, and I didn't need them. Of the two midwives who worked as a pair, this one was sympathetic to the situation of the past few weeks. She laughed and said, "Good for you." I was glad that she was on call; the other one seemed less supportive and found all the prenatal "problems," perhaps in an attempt to instill some fear and create a sense of dependency. She has more experience with birth and perhaps she's better educated to deal with emergencies, but I have more experience with me.

I knew my body best and I had faith in its ability to give birth. I knew that if the cord was around the baby's neck, I'd slip it off. I did not buy into the hysteria that infinite numbers of things could go wrong during birth. I believed it was more likely that everything would be just fine. I wanted complete responsibility for this baby. Some medical people will be horrified at my choice, but I felt that there were no immediate life and death reasons to justify a hospital. I decided that if something was so terribly wrong that my baby would not survive, I wanted to be the one to cradle it in my arms, in my opinion a far better way to pass on from this world than being poked, jabbed, and manhandled by people wanting appear heroic or wanting to avoid being sued. Babies arrive so vulnerable and helpless; more people need to stop and consider how they experience their first minutes of life. I believe that it does matter and it does make a difference to their perception of the world. Throughout my pregnancy, I felt that my baby was fine and I was confident that when the time came, my baby knew how to arrive in the world. Babies are far more intelligent than most people give them credit for being.

I was definitely on a hormone high. My son was perfect, and I felt great, aside from sitting down. Apparently I didn't need the midwife to "deliver" my baby. Who else but his mother would be sure he was handled with tender loving care? No brisk drying off with scratchy towels for this little person. No invasive tests. No slicing of his heel for a PKU test. No vitamin K. In the seconds immediately following birth, it didn't matter how much he weighed or how long he was, especially if knowing these details came at the expense of his sense of security and trust in the world as a safe place. He weighed what he weighed;

I would find out eventually. I held him exclusively for the first hours of his life. He was so small yet so strong.

I know I made the best choice for bringing this new soul into the world. A midwife may not like me, but I don't care! I am in love. I am the author of my own life.

∽

SHERA DANCER'S BIRTH STORY

I WAS AWAKENED Friday morning, January second, by Paco wanting to nurse. Nothing unusual; the day was beginning. I did notice cramps while lying in bed, but it was more the kind of feeling experienced before a bowel movement. Eventually Paco was ready to get up. After I had a bowel movement, my cramps did change. I felt this was prelabor, as the cramps were happening every so often and I felt them in my lower part. It definitely could not be labor: I was not expecting the baby for at least a few more days, really a week.

We planned to do our usual Friday stuff: get milk, eggs, and veggies, and we invited William over from across the street. Paco was very excited about playing more with William, so the three of us went for a good walk, exploring in the woods. I noticed the contractions seemed to have evened out somewhat. Previously they were happening frequently, when I got in and out of the car or made any unusual movement. During our walk, they seemed to calm down and spread out.

Paco went down for his nap, and I had lunch and wondered about this prelabor. It was getting pretty intense. I just had to stop through many contractions. I was thinking that I could not imagine many more days of this, and I was wondering when they would stop. Paco had a restless nap and woke up shortly after two o'clock, early for him. He nursed for a while, and I endured that, and then we just hung out, but I had to stop and breathe through contractions. This upset him. I would bend over with my hands on my knees, and he tried to get me up or just seemed upset.

I had cooked beans for hummus, so we went to work on that. I was sure that eventually these cramps would stop. Around three fifteen PM, I went to talk to Thomas, but he was pretty intent on what he was doing, so I said that I would come back in a bit. I continued to work in the kitchen, stopping and bending over regularly for contractions. A short while later, Thomas came in and I told him I was having contractions but that this was prelabor, nothing to worry about. He did not believe me and went to work getting the tub set up (but not filling it), bringing the bed downstairs, and going out to get some alcohol for placenta essence.

I continue on the hummus, cleaned the kitchen a bit, and then said, "Enough." I just needed to get inside myself more and concentrate on the contractions. Close to six PM, I decided that whether or not this labor was real, I wanted to be in the tub, so I asked Thomas to fill it. I was glad to get into the tub, though perhaps it was a bit warm. The contractions slowed, but I welcomed the break. In the other room I could hear Paco and Thomas eating their dinner, and occasionally one or both would come in to check on me.

After dinner Thomas called my sister, who lives an hour away. Paco had been bouncing off the walls all day, and Thomas was getting worn out. He figured he would need help getting Paco to sleep. I said jokingly that maybe the baby would be born by nine PM and I could help.

I had made many trips to the bathroom during the day. (It was important to me to continue peeing because with Paco's birth, I had a catheter because I could not pee.) At some point I was aware that I could no longer pee. I tried sitting on the toilet, squatting, using peppermint oil, letting go in the tub, but only a few drops would come out. It felt as if trying to pee brought on contractions, and if I tried to pee after a contraction, I still could not let go. I was starting to become concerned. I could feel my bladder and knew that emptying it would be helpful.

At some point I also accepted the idea that this must be real labor but wondered how I would survive many more hours. I asked Thomas, "Why am I doing this?" I checked myself: I did not know what I was feeling, but I did not feel too open, though way up I could feel something hard. It would be a long time yet. Thomas gave me a homeopathic remedy to see if that would help with peeing. Around eight PM, I told Thomas that if I had not peed by eight thirty, we would call the midwife.

Just before eight o'clock, we heard from my friend Tonya, whom Thomas had also called. She would be heading out soon. Just after eight, my sister called and said that she would also be heading out. I asked why we needed both of them. Thomas just shrugged. I went to the washroom again and felt I was pushing, felt that I was just pushing to pee but then told Thomas that I felt like I had to have a bowel movement.

When that contraction was over, I went to the kitchen. I had been drinking water with lemon but felt that some frozen juice would be good. I got the frozen juice out of the freezer, and Paco got his spoon to have some too. He was up on his chair, and we both dug in. Then the next contraction hit. (There was still a fair bit of time between many contractions, no regularity, but I was not timing them.) I yelled-growled and apologized to Paco, who went running away, scared by the intensity. I noticed that I was pushing. "Oh, no, I shouldn't be pushing yet!" Then I felt the baby move down, and she started to crown.

Thomas started to come toward me, and he noticed the head. At this point I felt it. He touched it, but I kept telling him not to touch it. I am pretty sure he took his hand off, but the intensity of the head half in is quite painful. I pushed again, and Thomas mentioned that the head was out and there were the shoulders. They came out on the next contraction with the rest of the baby along with her waters. She was born in the caul, with the amniotic sack still around her.

Thomas handed her to me as I was still standing and leaning on the back of Paco's chair. The baby was shrieking, and I was talking to her, trying to calm her down. I think I could have been gentler in my handling of her, but I was excited and shaking and thrilled to have a baby. Thomas grabbed the sheets to throw on the mess on the floor and put the chair underneath me to sit on. We figure that she came out around 8:27 PM. While I was sitting down, some blood gushed out of me, and since we did not have any shepherd's purse tea brewed, I chewed on the herb while the water was boiling. There was no problem with bleeding too much, but the scare that had been given to me about low hemoglobin and bleeding was somewhat noticeable. At some point I checked and saw that we had a girl! Yay! I was happy to have either sex, but deep down I had preferred a girl, although I had hardly dared to hope for that.

A few minutes later I lay down on the bed we had set up in the dining room. Ten minutes after the birth, Tonya showed up. I heard Thomas greeting her at the door with, "You're late!" My sister showed up around nine thirty PM. I am glad that they showed up after the birth. Tonya helped to keep me in liquids, and Olivia spent time playing with Paco. Paco had been looking on from the living room, whimpering as the baby was coming out. He did not want to go near her for at least a day, and bedtime was pretty distressing for him. It was after midnight by the time he fell asleep, exhausted, with me lying beside him, and the baby and her placenta on the other side of me.

Seventeen hours after her birth, we cut the cord, and six days later the stump fell off. She nursed shortly after birth and has been a nursing fiend almost ever since. The first day she hardly nursed at all as she slept most of it, and at ten days old she is still sleeping a lot.

It was a great birth. I feel so lucky to have a boy and a girl. We are still debating names. I guess we still have time, as I have to figure out all the paperwork for the birth certificate on my own now, with no midwife to do that for me.

⬡

IVY MCNIVEN'S BIRTH STORY

I LABORED AND birthed my children alongside my husband. He thinks it was just the two of us. I do not have the heart to tell him that a Wise Old Woman was there all along—he just could not see her or feel her. She called to me in every labor that I experienced, and by the time I was awaiting my last child, I looked forward to birthing with her again. My Wise Old Woman knew me, believed in me, respected me, and never judged me.

I heard her voice sooner and sooner with every labor, and off I would journey along a narrow mountain path overlooking the ocean. Sometimes I was afraid of losing my step and tumbling over the cliffside. Whenever I thought that I could not go on, I heard her voice calling me gently, echoing upward from the water's edge, her deep, loving sound filling me up inside.

When the mountain path ended, a slightly steep, tree-lined path opened up over the edge of the mountain, leading to the ocean. *Ah-h-h, it was time.* I always felt my body struggle desperately just before surrendering and stepping over the edge. I would climb downward while the trees appeared to shift their positions to support me when I needed extra help. All the while, my Wise Old Woman softly sang my name.

When I made it to the sandy, rocky ocean's edge, I followed her lovely voice while carefully picking my way around the giant rocks. She sat nestled inside a formation of stones that shielded her from the dark, churning ocean. She was always delighted to see me and always greeted me with outstretched arms. When I looked in her eyes, I knew I was loved unconditionally. She had a towering, strong body and long, dark, wild wavy hair. I would curl up in her arms, and she would sing to me about all the reasons I am worthy and all the times in my life I have expressed courage and strength. I would blurt out my fears or doubts, and she would simply sigh, "Ah-h-h, that's it. That's it!"

When the pounding waves grew stronger and louder and higher, she would gently push me away and tell me to help my baby. I would make my way out of the rocky shelter and squat and scream at the edge of the pounding waves while I birthed my baby.

Once I had birthed, I could hear my husband's voice again, and it would carry me back. He would cry out, "Way to go, sweetie. We did a great job!" I always smiled and gave him a thumbs up while closing my eyes—giving thanks—and trying to catch one last parting glimpse of my Wise Old Woman.

When I am challenged in my life, I can hear her words telling me how worthy and strong I am, and it fills me up. I do not miss her so much anymore now that I take her story and share it with other women.

"Ah-h-h, that's it. That's it."

MARY SIEVER'S BIRTH STORY

ABOUT SIX IN the morning on Monday, April ninth, I woke up briefly and felt a mild sensation like a contraction. At first I thought maybe it was just a gas pain, but when I had a couple more within a few minutes I realized it was not gas—it was a real contraction. Kim was half awake, and I told him that it looked like today might be the day.

We got up and started our day. Sinéad did not wake up immediately, so we left her in the bed, and I went to the kitchen to start breakfast. I made some pancakes and all the while mentally planned my day. I was getting excited. I realized this was probably really it, but because I was just beginning labor, it would not be right away.

Kim left for school, and I told him that I would keep him posted and that if the contractions got much stronger, I would tell him to get back home as soon as possible. I do think a solo birth is a really great idea, but it is not for me. I love having my husband there to be a strength, support, and comfort. It helps that he is so calm and knowledgeable about it, too.

I wanted to get some laundry finished, and I had to buy some more laundry soap. I also had two visiting teaching appointments. Sinéad and I headed out, and though she wanted to walk, I needed her to be in the stroller so I would not have to carry her because I did not feel up to that with waves of contractions coming every once in awhile. I wanted to walk as briskly as I could to keep things smooth. I noticed that not only did the contractions feel less intense when I was actually moving, but that moving does speed things up.

We went to our appointments, and on the way we saw several people who I knew would be surprised when they found out that our baby was to be born that day. We got home shortly before lunchtime, and I put Sinéad down for a nap. I nursed her, actually, which brought on some strong contractions. (Every little bit helps.) After this I phoned to arrange to pick up some birth supplies that were waiting for us. Kim was going to get them, and I needed the address. I e-mailed Kim the address and told him that he might want to think about coming home early.

I was starting to have to concentrate, and I tidied things up and did a bit of e-mailing. Sinéad slept until about one PM, and I got her up, fixed her some lunch, and started a bath for me. I was hoping Kim would be home soon but was not counting on it. I phoned the school, but just as I was trying to get a message to him, he pulled up in the driveway. As he came in the door, he told me that he had known he would be home early but wanted to surprise me.

I hopped in the bath, and Kim started to set things up downstairs for our planned water birth. Unfortunately, shortly after starting to fill the pool, he realized that it had a leak. Since all our stuff was downstairs—blankets, pillows, birth baskets, etc.—we were going to stay there, but I wanted to be near the tub, so Kim hauled everything back up—such a trooper! Sinéad was doing well the whole time. When I was vocalizing through some contractions, Kim told her that it meant the baby was coming, so every time she got a big grin on her face and said, "Baby coming!"

I found that being in the bath, moving around a lot—I "danced" through some contractions—and making low, strong sounds made a big difference, helping me to integrate the progression. When I had some especially intense contractions, I also talked to myself, which felt so good, and the self-talk made a difference too. Toward the end I squatted through some contractions, and that helped open me up and relieve the pressure. Around five PM, I came into the bedroom. Sinéad told Kim she wanted to lie down for a nap, so she was on the single bed we have next to our bed, and Kim covered her up.

I knelt against the end of the bed, and one very strong, intense contraction almost overcame me, but did not. It was an amazing contraction, and I could feel it opening me up. I am quite positive that I dilated fully at that point and that Regan moved down some more. Kim said, "Maybe you should get on the bed now." I did, as that was where all of our pads and things were located.

I knelt again, like I had done when I was birthing Sinéad, so far my favorite position to birth in. I concentrated on relaxing, and though I did not scream, I continued vocalizing through my contractions. A few minutes before six o'clock, my water broke during a contraction. I had a couple more contractions, and some more water came out. Kim had already started using the Crock-Pot to get the warm washcloths ready to support my perineum. I had asked him if it looked as though the head was coming, and he said, "Not yet, but you are really opening up." Even at this point, I figured I had a good couple of hours before the baby would be born.

That shows how much I knew. After the second splash of water came out, Kim was getting a washcloth, and I said, "The baby is coming!" Kim supported me again with the washcloths as I felt that ring of fire. The washcloths completely relieved the sensation. Another couple of contractions and I really had the urge to push. I had not truly felt that with Sinéad, but I sure could not help it with Regan. I did not give it everything I had, though; I let him ease out. His head emerged, and instead of pushing him right out, I waited for the next contraction. He slipped out, and though Sinéad was out of view to see the baby come out, she went out of the room and watched from the door. During the whole time, she showed no fear at all but curiosity and a good understanding. Regan did not have any mucus to cough up, and when Kim turned him over to rub his back to make sure, he complained rather loudly.

I turned onto my back and had Kim prop some pillows under my shoulders and back after taking Regan from him. We wrapped a towel around the baby, and though he did not nurse immediately, within a short while he did. Sinéad came up to see him and was very excited. We sat there for about an hour, and though I could feel that the placenta had separated within a couple of minutes, it did not come out. About forty-five minutes after Regan was born, Kim cut the cord and took him while I got up to squat over the bowl. I decided that I would rather sit on the toilet, so I went in there and pushed out the placenta.

After all this I realized how great I felt and still feel. I do not have the same soreness I had with Sinéad and no tearing, either. (I had a skid mark with Sinéad but no perineal tearing with her, either.) He is tinier than his sister was, nineteen inches long and weighing about six pounds. I am so thankful to my Heavenly Father for blessing us with this beautiful little boy.

Birthing naturally the first time or the next time

Reinekke Lengelle

There was a young woman,
who kicked off her shoes.
She had so many children by C-section
she knew what to do …

IT'S NO URBAN myth. After five caesarean sections, Kim Bisset went into labor, and when she was at the door, ready to be driven to the hospital with her midwife, she kicked off her boots and birthed him at home. She subsequently had two more babies at home with the help of a midwife. Sometimes this is the degree of faith and determination birthing requires, especially when the previous outcomes were undesired and disappointing.

To say that a woman who has given birth to a healthy baby should be glad regardless of the way the birth unfolded is a gross misunderstanding. Such a statement does not take into account that a woman may be legitimately grieving about the birth, quite apart from how she feels about the fruit of her labor. It also negates the fact that birth is a transition, a rite of passage that requires emotional adjustment even if the birth itself was uncomplicated.

As the stories in the previous chapters clearly show, birth cannot be predicted or scripted, and sometimes our experiences leave us with unprocessed pain and/or a longing to be more proactive in future pregnancies.

This chapter will discuss what you can do when a birth experience has left you unsatisfied and will show you how you can increase your chances of a positive birth outcome. It includes insight into current prenatal care, current labor and birth processes, and suggestions for the postpartum period.

⁓◦⁓

Preparing for the first or next birth

A WORD ON PRENATAL CARE: FACTS AND FICTION

How would you feel if you knew that the sugar in your urine during your first pregnancy was the placenta's way of demanding nourishment from the body and was really no cause for concern?[1] Or that your blood pressure rising at the end of pregnancy is more often than not associated with good outcomes and not likely to be a sign of a serious condition called preeclampsia?[2] And what if your hemoglobin sinking lower than your physician feels comfortable with is actually a perfect reflection of your blood volume rising in tandem with growing life within?[3]

If you're anything like me, you will feel relieved (and a little irked) to learn that many of the alarmist practices in prenatal care are based on rather dubious assumptions disguised as science. In fact, giving a pregnant woman a diagnosis like gestational diabetes or pregnancy-induced hypertension causes what the renowned obstetrician Dr. Michel Odent refers to as the "nocebo" effect: it robs an otherwise happy, healthy pregnant woman of her time to feel joyful and at ease.[4] With research now showing that stress hormones coursing through a mother's veins affect her baby, there are concrete reasons to counter that stress with knowledge and information.

If you're one of the more paranoid members of the natural birthing community, you could easily be convinced that a conspiracy exists to keep pregnant women within the confines of medically controlled birth. If you're less suspicious, you may at least find this information helpful to have. You may even consider printing relevant articles so you can present them to your caregiver; don't assume all caregivers are aware or knowledgeable just because they should be.[5]

~✎~

Caregivers

MY MIDWIFE SERVED me tea as I had my last little cry about the upcoming birth of my second child. My mother has likened the experience of anticipating birth to the feeling a sheep must have when it is being led to slaughter. While that metaphor wouldn't be my first choice, the idea does strike a cord: as women we go to a place where we may not have much control but must continue. With this in mind, it becomes even more apparent that the choice of caregiver is essential.

Recently a woman told me that she had chosen the family physician that her friends had recommended, but she did not like him. Instead of making a different choice (as she would do now), she went into labor, glad this particular physician was on vacation, and happily birthed her baby with the help of a nurse—a former midwife in her country of origin—who happened to be on that particular shift. The message here is: don't let your birth unfold by caregiver-default.

Also, when a caregiver that you trust completely and who supports your birth philosophy helps you make a decision that you had hoped you wouldn't be faced with, it softens the blow. It can also reduce the tendency to look back on the event and wonder if you made the right choice.

Even during the actual unfolding of labor, a sensitive caregiver can create opportunities for the woman (or couple) to begin the emotional adjustment to unexpected changes and interventions.

As with hiring a contractor to build our home or choosing a dentist whose quality and method of care we prefer, there is no shame in shopping around for a suitable caregiver. We may have liked our family physician's approach to treating our skin rash but find him or her incompatible with our philosophy and needs during pregnancy and childbirth. Remember that you are the client and can hire or fire your caregiver as you see fit.

~ঞ্চ~

The hospital trance

THE PSYCHOLOGIST FRITZ PERLS, founder of Gestalt therapy, once said that the deepest trance one will ever be in is the family trance. Because a trance is an altered state of awareness that focuses our attention in a particular way to the exclusion of other perspectives, it is essential to become aware of what our trance-triggers are and how they may affect us during pregnancy and birth. As family functioning is woven tightly against the backdrop of societal functioning (or dysfunctioning), it is important to also be aware of the beliefs that we have internalized from our culture and that have us responding in pre-programmed ways.

For instance, while home birth is still seen as the exception in North America, in other countries like The Netherlands, where I was born, it is considered a normal choice for a healthy pregnant woman. While I have been told here that I was "brave" to have a home birth, my girlfriends in The Netherlands would laugh at such a suggestion. What we deem normal, acceptable, or even safe may have more to do with a trance-like response to what we're hearing than an informed view.

Even the belief that we are likely to have a complicated birth because our mother and grandmother had one may well create a birth liability. In fact, we may have repeated this story to ourselves so often that it has become an entrancing mantra turned self-fulfilling prophecy. Adopting the attitude that the buck stops here can be useful. I remember my mother congratulating me for being one of the first women in our family in generations to birth without an episiotomy, an intervention I had read about, knew about, and intended to avoid.

Trances are powerful because they literally affect the way we birth and the way we believe we can birth. Recently I found this poignantly illustrated when a doula friend told me she was assisting a couple giving birth in hospital. They were well-prepared, well-informed, and determined to have their baby as naturally as possible. Both had advanced degrees and "high-powered" careers and were eager to learn about birth and how to avoid unnecessary interventions. Both had also been open to my friend's counsel about hospital procedures and their right to choose and question advice given by obstetrics unit staff.

Yet my friend saw an almost baffling shift take place when they entered the hospital. Instead of using what they had learned and prepared for, it was as if their good intentions and knowledge suddenly seemed to drop away and were replaced by a (perhaps deeper) need to give themselves over to the will of the so-called professionals. I concede that this is but one interpretation of what was happening for this couple, but I believe it may reflect a common authority-induced trance, in which medical staff may play a vital role. The mere whisper of such magic words as "it's better for the baby" induces a trance stronger than one produced by Pitocin.[6] Despite hopes for a natural birth, this couple, like many others, ended with a high-intervention birth.

A way to tell if you have indeed given away your power in this unconscious manner is if you wake up feeling like you have an emotional hangover.

It's important to note that we are all susceptible to trances. If the right trigger is present, we may forget ourselves and lose touch with the instincts and intuitions we can usually rely upon during the birthing process. I remember even a midwife telling me that while she helped her own daughter give birth at home, she heard a faint whisper from within saying "I want the best for her . . ." and became aware that the idea of the best was associated with hospital birth! She was shocked that she, too, held this deep-rooted cultural belief, especially after having helped hundreds of women to give birth at home.

A trance is like a spell and can only be broken by bringing our fears and beliefs into consciousness, just as the midwife did by listening to her own doubts and acknowledging their existence, thus allowing them to be released.

Writing out a list of beliefs we have about labor and birth, including those things we've been told, is a good way to unearth our preconceptions. In addition, by knowing what our default position may be in moments of fear or uncertainty, the grip of a trance's power may be loosened. This leaves us open to receive the messages that may bring to our attention real danger during birth and/or a genuine need for medical intervention.

Another empowering step in overcoming the doubts planted in our minds that induce mind-numbing trances is to find support for our deeply held wishes in circles that don't confirm our doubts, but instead shed light on and affirm other possibilities. Claudia Villeneuve, home birth mother after a caesarean explains:

> The moment I found out I was pregnant again, I knew that I did not want a second caesarean. I became so sure of this that when the OB said that I should prepare to lose my baby if I went ahead with the VBAC home birth, I realized how much smarter I was in the art of giving birth than she was with all her university degrees and years of medical experience. I knew then that not only I, but every woman, could dream the impossible dream of catching her baby all by herself. It was an epiphany for me. There was no fear in my heart, just hope.[7]

In other words, instead of submitting to the will and ideas of her obstetrician (which may well reflected this physician's medical-training-trance), Villeneuve researched giving birth vaginally after a caesarean[8] and found support for her "impossible dream." She later delivered beautifully at home in water. With a bit of faith, awareness, and good information, we can lift ourselves beyond the danger of giving our power to other, more official sounding voices.

Ultimately, the only trance that is useful and worthy of being in during the birthing process is the endorphin-induced trance that is a physiological fact of labor!

~∾~

Remember that you are a mammal

IN HIS BOOK and lectures, Dr. Michel Odent likes to point out that a most influential figure of our time was born in a stable among mammals. With inspiration from this story, we remember that we, too, are mammals and share similar needs, and at no time is this more apparent than when a woman is giving birth.

My mother lay on a cold hospital bed trying to give birth to baby number one. My sister-in-law put up with a gaggle of medical students at her first and second births. I spent a substantial part of my first daughter's birth avoiding medical interventions that loomed overhead and were mentioned with regularity. Three strikes right here. Dr. Odent would shake his head knowingly at these stories and simply explain that all these circumstances are counterproductive to normal physiological birth.

He even questions the fairly recent addition of men into the labor and delivery scene, though he concedes that hospitals often feel like unsafe environments to women, and in this capacity male partners and doulas may have a vital role to play. At a lecture Dr. Odent gave, egalitarian types like myself were slightly aghast at hearing this respected and experienced obstetrician question the value of a male partner's presence at birth. Yet when an obstetrical nurse piped up and said, "Yeah, doctor, what can we do about those darned men?" I was willing to believe that he was alluding to a possible problem.[9] So I asked if men who were present at birth could at least learn about the gravity of bringing life into the world, but Dr. Odent quickly shot my philosophy down. All idealism aside, he came right back to the basic question of what a woman needs during labor—not philosophically but physiologically.

The needs of a woman during labor are pretty basic, and during his lecture and workshop Dr. Odent summed them up several times: privacy, safety, warmth, and darkness. These needs are pretty much what she requires to get to sleep and what that will reduce the activity of the neocortex of the brain. For humans, birth is a mammalian event in which the primitive part of the brain must take center stage. When a woman feels watched, her neocortex is stimulated. When she is asked to answer questions like, "What is your address?" or "Have you had the strep B test?" her neocortex is stimulated. When the lights are bright and glaring, a cliché that lives on in hospitals everywhere, her neocortex is stimulated. If she feels threatened in any way, her labor simply slows so that, like a mammal, she can get up and find a safer place to have her baby.

Being surrounded by strangers is counter to the birthing woman's need for privacy. *Exit nurses, Dr. On-call, and white cloud of medical students.* Being surrounded by people to whom a woman may want to demonstrate her ability to labor naturally can trigger anxiety. *Exit mother, labor "coach," and friend with birth ideals.* Having people take videos or photos can also change the dynamics of birth, even if the woman herself asked for them before labor.

Some of the best birth outcomes Dr. Odent has studied come from a female health provider in Kobe, Japan, who in 300 births had only one perinatal death and one caesarean section. The women who birthed near her did so mostly alone in small darkened rooms. When she was asked to speak to midwives in Britain at Dr. Odent's invitation, this caregiver quite hilariously had nothing to teach, because her way of helping birthing women was notably devoid of activity and/or technique. She pretty much left them alone; a rare approach in our culture's perception of how a woman needs to be "supported" during birth.

To understand the resistance medical professionals often have to this non-interventionist approach, my father, Dr. J. J. T. Gerding,[10] presented me with a point of reflection:

> In our hectic society it is much more difficult to not do something than to take action of some kind. Someone who does nothing runs the risk of being blamed for negligence, whereas someone who intervenes looks like he/she is helping and can't be as easily reproached. That is a big problem.

Given the startling realization that when it comes to childbirth, less may be *a lot more*, it is not surprising that Dr. Odent suggests that the best resource for a laboring woman is a midwife who has had children herself and stays at a distance, quietly waiting for the birth to unfold. In fact he says, "If you have found a midwife, I am useless." In London, where Dr. Odent works with a doula, he says he practically hides during labor so there is little or no presence (read: interference) at the birth. He and this doula provide three-day information sessions on birthing to mothers and grandmothers, and the only prerequisite for admission to the program is: "Who is the doula and what is the quality of her heart?" He overtly states that these information sessions are not about "training" a caregiver; instead the focus remains on who the doula is, not what she does.

～

Is birth like sex?

I'VE HEARD IT said that the environment in which a child is born should be similar to that in which the child was conceived. In reflecting on that, I thought about some ways in which making love does indeed mirror the conditions we envision for a natural birth. Though some of the following points are made tongue in cheek, they are worth a thoughtful laugh!

- You are safe and have privacy while doing it.
- You can move around and change positions often.

- You can soak in hot water and have candles burning.
- You can stay put when things get active.
- You can lose your mind. (Read: neocortical activity)
- You don't have to put up with unnecessary interventions.
- You can do what your body wants to.
- You don't get frozen from the waist down.
- You can make as much noise as you want to without feeling embarrassed.
- There are no strange germs!
- You might be a bit sore afterward, but you're allowed to walk around.
- You'll probably look radiant afterward.
- Everything will be done with your consent.
- You'll feel a high point near the end.
- Your partner is your main squeeze.
- You can go to sleep right afterward.

Keeping everything in the pie

IN MANY BOOKS about childbirth, including this one, you will be encouraged to make a birth plan. This can be a useful step in focusing your intent and communicating how you would like to be supported by those who will be involved as you give birth. On the other hand, having a birth plan doesn't mean that the birth will go as planned. In fact, the term may rightly be viewed as an oxymoron and might better be replaced by a term such as "plan of care for the birth."[11]

In preparing for my second birth, five years after my first, I took a course called Birthing from Within.[12] In one of its unusual sessions it was explained that birthing options and outcomes might be compared to the pieces in a pie, with each piece representing an event, intervention, or outcome we may be faced with regardless of our hopes and expectations. The problem with leaving out an option (for instance, deciding to refuse a caesarean section under almost any circumstance) is that if we are faced with this outcome, we will have a doubly hard time coming to terms with the birth afterward. Or, as the truism goes, expectations will get you into trouble every time. By allowing each piece to remain in the pie, while being well-informed and having a positive intention, we prepare ourselves for birth in a way that is truly unconditional. We may still want a natural vaginal birth, but we will be better able to deal with one that includes an epidural—a choice we didn't make lightly.

In hindsight, I could see the usefulness of the pie metaphor. My first birth had unfolded quite differently than I had planned. In fact, my first daughter, Sophia, was born with the help of an epidural and other painkilling drugs in a hospital instead of at home where I had hoped she would come into the world. What killed my joy, more than the experience itself, was that I had so vehemently rejected the acceptability of an epidural beforehand and as a result found it hard to forgive myself for the choices I made during her birth.

I have also found that internalizing the values that accompany a desire for natural childbirth can be a double-edged sword. The upside is the empowered choices one is able to make on the life-giving journey of pregnancy and birth. The downside is that self-criticism can creep in when these good intentions turn to dashed hopes. Though the values promoting natural birth are worthy and important, if we turn them on others and on ourselves as irrefutable laws, we can do damage while ignoring the varying circumstances and experiences that birthing women face.

For instance, I remember an advocate of natural birth who spoke very negatively about the epidural, questioning the need for it. Juxtaposed with this was her own revelation that she had had her own child in under two hours from first contraction to the baby's actual appearance into the world. Though I believe that the rate of epidural anesthesia could be greatly reduced in North America, I felt the need to come to the defense of women like myself who had labored for more than two days and opted for this intervention.

Interestingly, in her book *Women's Bodies, Women's Wisdom,* Christiane Northrup, a physician, determined that women who are too fixed on desired birth outcomes can create the opposite effect and actually end up with more medical interventions. This can be likened to the hang-glider who doesn't want to hit a building or post upon landing but does so precisely because his gaze is focused on it.

❧

Dealing with fears: it's an art

There are a lot of fears associated with birthing in our culture, and clearly they can't always be remedied by having correct information or feeling confident about our goal to birth naturally. Sometimes we need to look to subtler, less linear ways of coming to terms with our preconceptions and anxiety. I learned this at one of my Birthing from Within[13] classes when we were asked to create birth art.

The instructions were not to speak but to close our eyes and allow an image or thought to come up that revealed a fear we had around a certain aspect of our upcoming birth. I closed my eyes and quite unexpectedly saw an image of my baby with the cord around the neck. I dismissed it as a stereotypical fear but drew it anyway. Without speaking we were asked to flip our picture over and draw the solution on the other side. I drew the midwife correcting the problem and wrote "competent caregiver" beside the drawing. I never gave this exercise another thought and felt no cause for concern. My daughter Maya was indeed born with the cord around her neck (not once but twice) and our midwife unwrapped it with lightening speed. My artistic portrayal of events and the spontaneous inner vision I'd had proved to be more fact than fiction.

Interestingly, I had also wanted to know the gender of our baby before she was born but after a bit of deliberation decided I would wait. During the week of my intense deliberations, I dreamed that an ultrasound technician told me we were going to have another girl. That, too, came true. Ironically, I had no ultrasounds done during either of my pregnancies.

Ultimately, I believe these poignant experiences tell us that our inner resources for knowing and overcoming fear are richer than we are taught to believe.

❧

Asking for what you need and expressing feelings

BEING A WOMAN of the twenty-first century, you should know what you want and ask for it, right?

Wouldn't it nice if we were so in tune every moment and so lacking in inhibitions that when we give birth we could tell those present what we need so that our labor might be easier and less complicated? Allowing yourself to change your mind and/or to speak your body's language based on loud or subtle impulses during labor may be necessity rather than luxury.

Though I hope we've progressed beyond the era when women internalized messages like "if you can't say anything nice, don't say anything at all," we may need to reaffirm our commitment to asking for what we need, thereby allowing ourselves autonomy over the experience. If you want that in plain language: try being selfish during labor. It may be one of the only times you feel justified in getting away with it so fully, and in the process you're doing everyone involved a favor!

On the day I went into labor with my second daughter, my friend Marlene arrived to be with us and help me through the process. We spent the day together but by late evening, both of us got the sense that something was stalling my labor. My husband and I went for a walk and on returning home I sat down and told Marlene that I felt embarrassed knowing that she would see me in such a primal state. Since she had given birth twice herself and is a friend who knows me well, her empathetic listening felt genuine and reassuring and I was able to go into labor in front of her. Within an hour of that conversation labor began strongly, and eight hours later Maya was born.

Whether it is something as emotionally tender as this or whether it is as simple as asking the midwife and spouse to leave the bathroom when you need to use it, asking for what you need in each moment of labor helps the process unfold. Essentially you are asking for and affirming your need for those key physiological conditions that will help labor to progress without unnecessary barriers.

~~~&~~~

Your partner

I bought a Superman T-shirt for my husband after the birth of our second daughter. This was the only macho gesture that became part of Maya's birth history. He had earned this not by leaping over buildings in single bounds but by a few other heroic deeds, not the least of which was massaging me for hours with hands of steel and holding my full pregnant weight up just before the crowning. More than anything, his ability to respond to what I asked for during labor and the surrender to his duty as self-professed (S)erf was what earned him this badge of honor.

In preparing this chapter, I asked one of my sisters what she most needed in preparation for birth. She told me she had asked her husband to read to her during labor and tell her to relax often. Predictably there was a point in the labor process at which she asked him to put the book away, but she continued to benefit tremendously from his tender voice telling her to relax at every contraction. While some women would not respond kindly to being told to relax during labor *by anyone*, this was what worked for them and stemmed from a prelabor dialogue and from my sister anticipating her unique needs.

Although I've mentioned Dr. Michel Odent's view on men present at a birth, I have also heard (and this book contains numerous illustrations) of how a partner or husband can be a welcome and nurturing presence at a birth. It seems that the success of support offered by our partner is greatly influenced by our established relationship, our ability to communicate our needs, and our partner's willingness to take cues from us. Dr. John Gottman, a marriage expert, even says that a man's overall willingness to "take influence" from his wife a vital indicator as to whether or not the relationship will last.

Last, it is no small asset for a man (or birth partner) to understand what natural physiological birth looks like and to leave the birthing woman in "laborland."[14] This was nicely illustrated by a story of a woman who while in labor rolled her eyes back into her head so far that her husband became concerned about her. When he remembered that during birth he may see her in ways he wasn't used to, he calmed himself and allowed her to stay in her state of sheer concentration, and did not stimulate her neocortex by alarming her and setting off a process of "adrenaline contagion."[15]

∽❧∾

The postpartum period: healing processes

Imagine yourself in your home a few days after birth. You are nursing your newborn and for the most part you're healing: physically that is. Yet on some almost intangible level you feel that the birth itself was a kind of violation. Your partner says it all went remarkably well and reaffirms that you were a true birth warrior and that the baby looks great.

You can't quite put your finger on it....

Was it the way the obstetrician tried to pry you open and left fingerprints on the baby's tender scalp that is upsetting? Is it the fact that you must now tell your friends that you went for the drugs when you'd sworn you wouldn't? Or could it be the way you looked when you first saw yourself in the mirror after forced pushing encouraged by a labor coach disguised as a nurse? Or is it the thought that you were naked and moaning when three interns walked in?

In some respects, birth is part of what happens to us while we're busy making other plans. Naomi Wolf, author of *Misconceptions*, mentioned on *Oprah* that she was appalled that her caesarean birth left her feeling like she had been hit by a truck. Other women have expressed being disappointed and dejected or even feeling abused during and after the experience of giving birth. They find themselves angry with their physicians, their partners, God, and sometimes even with their own babies.

Some women have described the feeling of being half dead as a result of the epidural anesthesia. In fact, a sense of disembodiment along with feelings of being traumatized, humiliated, or filled with self-blame are common, and I'm not referring to postpartum depression here. (Or perhaps a lesser-known cause of postpartum depression is related to how a woman was treated while she birthed. I believe this is an area worthy of further research.)

In an attempt to acknowledge the beauty of birth, one might suggest that we should be in awe of this magnificent, miraculous event. Yet maybe it is in part these idealistic-sounding terms that leave us so unprepared for the rawness and intensity of this life-giving journey. I've heard a doula say, "Please don't use the term gentle when you talk about birth. We can treat a woman in labor and the baby with gentleness, but birth is hard work physically and emotionally."

OTHERS' STORIES THAT HEAL

In a culture where babies are welcomed with sentimental cards and parties where the well-meaning emphasis is often on gift giving in the material sense, there may be a lack of meaningful celebrations and a need instead to be "showered" with real and encouraging stories. Yet birth stories shared in conversation are often filled with accounts of pain, horror, and more recently drugs.

Only by reading and hearing stories considered "alternative" do we remember what birth might otherwise be like. In the end, I believe hearing many stories about the process and outcome of birth with the intention of sharing and informing can help reshape the way we view this natural process. By knowing the stories of other women, as we do in this collection, we can also see that each experience is unique and imperfect in its own way and we may find ourselves remembering our own experiences in a more balanced and forgiving manner.

Others' birth stories can help us to bridge the transition into motherhood, as it affects us all in physical, emotional, psychological, and even spiritual ways.

WRITING IT OUT

As a writer, I often reach for my pen when I have unprocessed grief or pain, but when it came to writing the story of Sophia's birth I waited a full year. I also bled for a year after her birth and miraculously stopped bleeding the day I wrote down our story. Like a spell in a fairy tale broken by naming the name, the healing began.

I could tell you that it was a lack of time that kept me from writing, but more truthfully I was trapped in my own shame and as yet unprepared to break through it. An unspoken and unexplored question lay at the foundation of my inability to go to the page for comfort and resolution. The question sounded something like: "Won't writing this story just add insult to injury? Now you will not only have failed at birth, but you will have to say so on the page as well." It was too much to bear.

When I finally did write the story, I wrote not only about the event but also about the feelings surrounding the birth. According to Dr. James W. Pennebaker, a professor at the University of Texas and a renowned researcher on the connection between health and emotional disclosure, writing about both events and feelings associated with them is precisely the combination that promotes healing. (My writing session ended with a very good cry over the keyboard!)

Though I had long believed in the unity of mind and body in health, it didn't really sink in until I experienced actual physical healing. I believe my body was crying for me by bleeding, and by allowing myself to grieve instead, I took the onus off the body and it was able to restore itself.

Letting all our "voices" be heard

Realizing that we can remember our experience of giving birth with a multitude of mixed feelings and not a consistent, unchanging story can take away the sting of a single conclusion. For instance, one part of you may feel relieved about the birth; another part may give you a failing grade; while a third aspect is heard saying, "It is as it is; be kind to yourself." By listening and recording these divergent voices, I have found that the stressful black or white thinking around our experience starts to shift. The realization that we can feel all these contradictory things simultaneously can even be humorous and refreshing. In various psychological streams these many voices are sometimes referred to as sub-personalities or sub-satellites and can be likened to the various actors on the stage of life, each actor reflecting a part of ourselves, exploring and expressing our drama and wisdom.[16] I have used this process in dealing with a miscarriage, literally writing out what each inner character had to say and finding that there were parts of me that fully accepted the "loss" as it unfolded.[17] I emotionally (and literally) came "to terms" with the miscarriage by allowing the variety of my reactions to be expressed.

ASKING TOUGH QUESTIONS
AND FINDING GENTLE ANSWERS

I once recounted the story of Sophia's birth to a friend about four months afterward. He must have sensed my need to defend myself and wryly commented, "So that's your story and you're sticking by it, are you?" This irked me somewhat, and I now realize that we can easily get trapped in our own version of what happened. In questioning whether our presumptions about our performance and the event are really as true as we try to convince ourselves they are, specific self-directed questions can be useful. I have found the four-question inquiry process by Byron Katie very helpful. "Who would you be without your story?" is a question that her process revolves around. Imagine that you are thinking "I could have done better" but by truthfully feeling the answer to a simple question like "Is it true?" or "Can you absolutely know that it's true (that you could have done better)?" you realize, without rationalizing, that you did the best you could at the time. Answering even just these first two questions of her process may be enough to free us of our mental torture.[18]

In hindsight I see that I experienced more pain from my own thinking about Sophia's birth than from the actual days I spent in labor. Or as Shakespeare wrote, "There is nothing either good or bad, but thinking makes it so."

I realize at the completion of this chapter that I could have spoken about many other aspects of birth and ways to prepare (i.e., hypnosis, visualization, options in prenatal education), but I chose to focus on subjects I felt are not typically considered in mainstream publications about pregnancy and birth. For that I am particularly indebted and grateful to Dr. Michel Odent and Pam England.

I toyed with the idea of including the words "uncommon wisdom" in my chapter title but hope instead that what I've shared sounds like common sense.

My experiences with birth have shown me that preparation—not just on a physical level—pays off. While my first birth experience was difficult and left me feeling bereft, I can look back on my second birth experience with joy. The pain of labor and my efforts to bring my daughters into the world were not so different, but what was different was the way I felt about myself, about the care I received, and about the way my body was able to do its work.

In summary: don't be taken in by the widespread fear mongering of the medical community, when it comes to prenatal care as well as labor and birth processes. Get informed, rely on your instincts, and dispel beliefs that leave you vulnerable to trances. Choose your caregiver(s) with heartfelt conviction, bring them up-to-date information, and make sure you and your caregiver(s) have a solid understanding of your physiological needs during labor. Remember also that birth unfolds beyond our control, though the conditions that facilitate the likelihood of a more natural birth can be created. If you've had a birth that has left you with a sense of regret or disappointment, know that you can heal through the stories of others and the tone and quality of the story that you tell yourself.

Finally, I wish you a birth you can look back on with joy.

REINEKKE LENGELLE has an MA in Adult Education from the University of Leiden, The Netherlands. She is a published playwright, poet, and self-help author and has written many magazine articles. She spent three years as a writer-in-residence for the award-winning Artists-on-the-Wards program at the University of Alberta Hospital and has designed and taught many inspirational writing courses. She has also served as a magazine editor for *Birth Issues* and is currently an assistant professor with Athabasca University: Canada's Open University.

Glossary

⌐

ADRENALINE (EPINEPHRINE): Hormone produced by the adrenal glands; commonly known as the fight/flight hormone, it causes an increase in blood pressure, heart rate, aggressiveness, and anxiety; an antagonist to oxytocin.

AFTERBIRTH: See *placenta*.

AFTERPAIN: Contractions of the uterus in the postpartum period; often felt during breastfeeding.

AMNIOTIC FLUID: Fluid surrounding the fetus in the uterus.

AMNIOTIC SAC: Membranes surrounding the fetus while in the uterus; filled with amniotic fluid, it is commonly known as the bag of waters.

AMNIOCENTESIS: Prenatal test involving removal and analysis of a small amount of amniotic fluid from the uterus in order to detect congenital abnormalities or the level of maturation of the fetus.

AMNIOTOMY: Surgical rupture of membranes; AROM; commonly known as breaking the water.

ANALGESICS: Medications that reduce pain.

ANESTHETIC: Medication that blocks sensation locally or generally; also induces muscle relaxation.

ANTERIOR POSITION (OCCIPUT ANTERIOR): Baby's position in the uterus where the back of the baby's head is toward the front of its mother.

APGAR SCALE: General test of newborn immediately after birth that checks heart rate, breathing, circulation, responsiveness, and muscle tone, scoring in the range 0 to 10 (a score of 8 to 10 indicates a newborn in good condition).

AUGMENTATION (OF LABOR): The use of synthetic hormones to supplement the natural contractions in labor, often heightening the intensity and pain of contractions leading to increased use of analgesics/epidural anesthesia and other interventions.

BACH FLOWER REMEDIES: Discovered by Dr. Bach, thirty-eight remedies made from plant/flower essences that can positively affect one's emotional state.

BIRTH CANAL: *See* vagina.

BIRTH CENTER: Independent or free-standing home-like alternative to a hospital, where women can choose to give birth.

BIRTH PLAN (PLAN OF CARE FOR THE BIRTH): Document prepared by the expectant woman or couple that outlines choices they have made about their care during childbirth and which they would like to see respected.

BIRTHING BALL: Large inflated ball on which the woman can sit or lean to ease the discomfort of labor and allow her to be supported when she moves into different positions during the birthing process.

BIRTHING STOOL: Short stool on which a woman can sit or bear down during labor, designed with an open front so that the baby can be born while the woman remains on the stool.

BLOODY SHOW: Normal, blood-tinged mucus secretions from the vagina as a result of cervical effacement and dilation.

BRADLEY METHOD: Childbirth preparation method that relies on "coaching" or support provided by the partner of the laboring woman; intended to facilitate natural childbirth.

BRAXTON HICKS CONTRACTIONS: Light and painless tightenings of the uterus that happen during gestation and are often not felt until the end of pregnancy.

BREECH PRESENTATION: Position in which the baby lies with buttocks or feet down rather than with the head down; three types include complete, Frank, and footling.

BORN IN THE CAUL: When the baby is born with an intact amniotic sac; the sac bursts or is artificially ruptured so that the baby can breathe. In old folklore, a caul birth was seen as good luck, especially for sailors.

CD: Certified doula.

CAESAREAN/C-SECTION: Major abdominal surgery in which a baby is removed through an incision made in the abdominal and uterine wall.

CAUL: *See* born in the caul.

CEPHALIC PRESENTATION: Position in which the baby lies with the head down; four types include vertex, military, brow, and face.

CERVIX: Neck of the uterus that extends into the vagina; the opening is termed the os.

CHROMOSOMAL ABNORMALITY: Genetic abnormality that shows up on the set of 23 chromosomes (rod-like structures containing genetic information); may be detected through invasive prenatal tests.

CNM: Certified nurse midwife.

CONCEPTION: Fertilization of the egg by the sperm and its subsequent implantation in the uterine wall.

CONTRACTION: Tightening of the uterus in (regular) intervals to facilitate the dilation of the cervix and press the baby through the birth canal.

CPM: Certified professional midwife.

CROWNING: Moment when the baby's head appears at the opening of the vagina and does not slip back inside; the sensation for the mother is likened to a "ring of fire."

DECELERATIONS: Periodic drop in the fetal heart rate; does not necessarily indicate distress of the fetus.

DEMEROL: A derivative of morphine. *See* analgesics.

DILATION: Opening of the cervix during labor, usually measured in centimeters (10 cm referring to fully dilated).

DONA: Acronym for Doulas of North America; as of 2004 this organization is called DONA International.

DOPPLER: An electronic listening device for monitoring the fetal heart rate.

DOULA: Greek word that has come to mean a woman experienced in childbirth and professionally trained to provide physical, emotional, and informational support during pregnancy, labor, birth, and the immediate postpartum period.

DOWN'S SYNDROME: Chromosomal abnormality (trisomy 21) that leads to mental retardation and physical malfunctions; many babies with this condition can survive and grow to adulthood with medical care.

DYSTOCIA: Difficult labor due to the positioning of the baby in the pelvis or ineffective uterine contractions.

ECLAMPSIA: Severe condition which can occur during pregnancy, in labor or within 48 hours of childbirth with symptoms similar to preeclampsia.

EDD/EDB: Estimated due date/estimated date of birth.

EFFACEMENT: Softening of the cervix measured in percentages, 100 percent being fully effaced.

ENGAGEMENT: When the baby's presenting part is deep in the mother's pelvic cavity, which often happens near the end of pregnancy.

EPIDURAL ANESTHESIA (LUMBAR EPIDURAL BLOCK): Combination of an anesthetic and a narcotic agent injected into the extradural space of the lower spine to block out labor pain and/or to prepare for a caesarean.

EPISIOTOMY: Cut made in the perineum from the vaginal opening toward the anus, intended to help speed delivery; research has shown that an episiotomy heals more slowly and causes more complications than a tear as well as increasing sevenfold the woman's chances of getting a fourth-degree tear (a tear through the anal sphincter).

ENDORPHINS: Opiate-like protein secreted naturally by the body (during labor) to raise pain tolerance and produce sedation and euphoria; use of narcotic analgesics such as Demerol and morphine can interfere with a birthing woman's natural endorphin release, thereby reducing her ability to cope naturally.

FALSE LABOR: Contractions that mimic real labor but are not. *See* Braxton Hicks contractions.

FETAL DISTRESS: Impaired fetal circulation during birth; indicated by a change in fetal heart rate. *See* fetal tachycardia and decelerations.

FHR: Fetal heart rate.

EFM: Electronic fetal monitoring: continuous monitoring of the fetal heart rate with a Doppler device, either strapped to the woman's belly or with a handheld device (used externally and continuously or intermittently) or through an electrode inserted into the baby's scalp (internal) while in the birth canal.

FETAL PRESENTATION: The part of the fetus that enters the pelvic cavity first: cephalic (head), shoulder, breech.

FETAL TACHYCARDIA: High fetal heart rate of 160 beats or more per minute noted continuously for ten minutes via electronic fetal monitoring; can be related to epidural induced fever in the mother.

FETUS: Baby in utero between the twelfth week of pregnancy and birth.

FORCEPS: Metal spoon-like obstetrical instrument used to pull the baby out of the birth canal.

FUNDUS: Upper part of the uterus.

GESTATION: Pregnancy: the time between conception and birth.

GESTATIONAL DIABETES: Transitory change in the processing of carbohydrates during pregnancy that can be remedied by the reduction of simple carbohydrates (sugars) in the diet and increased exercise.

GBS: Prenatal test done late in pregnancy to detect if the normal flora of the vagina includes the presence of group B streptococcal bacteria; a positive test result would mean the woman may decide to receive IV antibiotic treatment during labor.

HEMOGLOBIN: Oxygen-carrying substance in the red blood cells containing iron.

HOMEOPATHICS: Therapies whereby minute amounts of a remedy that would usually cause symptoms are administered to treat those same symptoms.

HORMONE: Chemical naturally produced by the tissues, organs, or glands that has specific regulatory effects on another part of the body.

HYPNOBIRTHING: Childbirth preparation method employing deep relaxation, slow breathing patterns, and self-guided release of endorphins, with the aim of enabling a woman to experience natural childbirth.

INDUCTION (OF LABOR): Process of initiating labor using natural, pharmaceutical, or surgical means.

INFORMED CONSENT: Legal term defining a person's right to autonomy and self-determination whereby the woman must have the legal capacity, an understanding of proposed procedure (its risks, benefits, and alternatives), and makes a decision free of coercion about whether or not to allow the proposed procedure.

IV: Intravenous: injection of a drug and/or fluid directly into the bloodstream.

JAUNDICE (PHYSIOLOGIC): A common condition of newborns, caused by the inability of the liver to break down excess red blood cells, resulting in yellow pigmentation of the skin; can be remedied by exposure to direct light; usually harmless and disappears within two weeks of birth.

KEGEL EXERCISES: Muscle-tightening exercises for the perineum.

LABOR: The process of childbirth from the start of contractions to the birth of the baby and the placenta. Stage 1: dilation and effacement of the cervix; stage 2: full dilation to the birth of the baby; stage 3: the delivery of the placenta.

LAMAZE METHOD: Method of preparing for birth based on breathing techniques, also known as psychoprophylaxis; intended to promote natural childbirth.

LITHOTOMY: Position for birth in which the mother lies flat on her back with her legs wide apart in stirrups; the most common position for birth in the hospital is a modified lithotomy where the head of the bed is raised slightly (which actually interferes with delivery by decreasing the size of the pelvic opening).

MECONIUM: First contents of the bowel in the fetus, blackish-green in color; when present in the amniotic fluid before delivery may indicate fetal distress.

MIDWIFE: Practitioner of midwifery; provides care and advice to women and their families during pregnancy, labor, and the postpartum period; provides newborn care, breastfeeding support, and attends births on her own responsibility; practices in hospitals, clinics, health units, birth centers, or homes and is a specialist in normal childbearing. Midwives see childbearing as a normal life process, use minimal intervention, foster women's responsibility for their own health, have a holistic view of health, and support informed choice and continuity of care.

MISCARRIAGE (SPONTANEOUS ABORTION): Loss of pregnancy before the twentieth week of gestation.

MOLDING: Shaping of the baby's head to accommodate its passage through the birth canal during labor.

MORPHINE: Derivative of narcotic opium used as an analgesic.

MUCUS PLUG: Collection of thick mucus that plugs the cervical opening during pregnancy; the loss of this plug is a sign of impending labor.

NARCOTICS: Opiate drugs that induce a state of stupor. *See* analgesics.

NATURAL CHILDBIRTH: Labor and delivery without pharmaceutical, surgical, and/or other medical interventions.

NOCEBO EFFECT: Term coined by the obstetrician/midwife Michel Odent in which a patient (mother) is given information about her health that induces stress and has a negative effect on her well-being during pregnancy (opposite of a placebo).

NUCHAL CORD: Umbilical cord wrapped around the baby's neck.

OB/GYN: Obstetrician/gynecologist: a physician/surgeon specializing in the medical management of pregnancy, childbirth, and female health.

OXYTOCIN: Naturally occurring hormone involved in labor, breastfeeding, and orgasm; having both physical and emotional effects. Also referred to as the "hormone of love."

PERINEUM: Area between and around the vagina and the anus.

PIH: Pregnancy induced hypertension (high blood pressure).

PITOCIN/SYNTOCINON: Synthetic hormone used to induce or augment labor and/or speed delivery of the placenta; designed to mimic the physical effects of oxytocin but does not cross the blood/brain barrier as oxytocin does; cannot replicate the positive emotional effects of natural childbirth.

PLACENTA: Organ that is implanted in the wall of the uterus and provides the baby with nourishment through the umbilical cord; it is delivered after the baby in the third stage of labor.

POSTPARTUM: Period following birth.

POSTPARTUM HEMORRHAGE: Excessive bleeding (more than 500 ml) from uterus after the birth.

POSTTERM: A pregnancy that lasts longer than forty-two weeks.

POSTERIOR (OCCIPUT POSTERIOR): Baby's position in the uterus where the baby's head (crown) is toward the mother's back.

PREECLAMPSIA: Condition during pregnancy where a woman has high blood pressure, water retention, protein in the urine, and often excessive weight gain; also known as toxemia.

PROLAPSED CORD: When the umbilical cord enters the birth canal before the baby does; if the baby's head is engaged prior to the rupture of the membranes, this condition is unlikely.

PRECIPITOUS LABOR: Rapid progression of labor and birth.

PREMATURE/PRETERM: Baby born before the thirty-seventh week of pregnancy.

QUICKENING: First fetal movements felt by the mother; usually experienced between sixteen and nineteen weeks' gestation, sometimes earlier.

RELAXIN: Protein secreted by the ovaries that relaxes the pelvic joints in late pregnancy and is a factor in initiating dilation of the cervix.

RM: Registered midwife.

RN: Registered nurse.

SAC: See *amniotic sac.*

STILLBIRTH: Birth of a dead baby.

TEAR: Laceration of the perineum; measured by degree ranging from 1 to 4 (1 being minor: not requiring suturing, 4 being a major tear through the anal sphincter: requiring careful surgical repair).

TENS: Transcutaneous (via the skin) electronic nerve stimulation: used to naturally induce labor and as a natural pain-coping tool.

TERM: Baby born between thirty-seven and forty-two weeks' gestation.

TRADITIONAL BIRTH ATTENDANT: A woman who provides prenatal care and attends to birthing women but has no professional designation; also known as a lay midwife.

TRANCE: Focusing of the mind in a particular way to the exclusion of other ways; a trance makes us vulnerable to suggestion, coercion, or denial, filtering out possibly relevant information.

TRANSITION: Period in labor when the woman dilates between from seven to ten centimeters between the first and second stages of labor; often the period of most pain due to the intensity and frequency of contractions.

TRIMESTER: Three-month period in pregnancy, of which there are three in total ("fourth trimester" is a term sometimes used to refer to the first three months of the postpartum period).

TRISOMY 18: Chromosomal abnormality causing multiple physical and mental conditions and deformities; babies rarely survive beyond forty-eight hours.

ULTRASOUND: Prenatal diagnostic tests (scan) made during pregnancy by a technician or physician of the fetus and/or other contents of the uterus.

UMBILICAL CORD: Cord that houses the blood vessels between the fetus and the placenta; this connection between maternal and fetal circulation provides the nourishment for fetal development.

UNASSISTED/UNATTENDED BIRTH: Birth where no trained caregiver (midwife, physician, or traditional birth attendant) is present.

UTERUS (WOMB): Hollow muscular organ in which the fetus develops from conception onward.

VACUUM EXTRACTION: Alternative to forceps delivery where the baby is removed from the birth canal by suction while the mother bears down.

VAGINA: Canal between the uterus and the external genitals (vulva).

VBAC: Vaginal birth after caesarean.

VERSION (EXTERNAL/INTERNAL): Turning a breech presentation to a cephalic presentation.

WATER BIRTH: Birth where the mother uses submersion in water as a pain-coping measure and where the baby is born under water.

Notes

~

INTRODUCTION

1 André Picard, 2004, "Natural birth no longer the norm in Canada," *Globe and Mail*, (September)10: A-11.

2 Gail Johnson, 2004, "C-section debate cuts both ways," *Straight.com* 11 (March), <http://www.straight.com/content.cfm?id=1357>.

3 Maternity Wise Web site <http://www.maternitywise.org/mw/aboutmw/index.html ?hormones>.

4 Marsden Wagner, 1998, "Midwifery in the industrialized world." *Journal of the Society of Obstetricians and Gynaecologists of Canada*, (November). Reprinted in *Birth Issues* magazine and available on-line at <http://www.asac.ab.ca/BI_fall99/midwifery.html>.

BIRTHING NATURALLY WITH A MIDWIFE

1 International Confederation of Midwives (ICM), *International Definition of the Midwife*, <http://www.internationalmidwives.org/Statements/Definition%20of%20the%20 Midwife.htm>.

2, 18 Odent, M. *The Farmer and the Obstetrician*. London: Free Association Books, 2002.

3 Alberta Association of Midwives (AAM) <http://www.albertamidwives.com>.

4, 10 *Midwifery in Alberta.* AAM, 1996. [video]

5 *Giving Birth: Challenges and Choices.* (Professional version with teaching guide). S. Arms, 1998. [video]

6 ASAC. *Planning for Birth.* Edmonton: ASAC, 2000. [booklet]

7, 13 Alberta Health and Wellness Workforce Planning Branch. *Midwifery Standards of Competency and Practice*, 1994.

8, 11, 19 Kitzinger, S. *Rediscovering Birth.* London: Little, Brown, 2000.

9, 17 Marsden Wagner, 1998, "Midwifery in the industrialized world." *Journal of the Society of Obstetricians and Gynaecologists of Canada*, (November). Reprinted in *Birth Issues* magazine and available on-line at <http://www.asac.ab.ca/BI_fall99/midwifery.html>.

10, 12 Canadian Association of Midwives (CAM). Position statement: Home birth <http://www.members.rogers.com/canadianmidwives> March 2001.

14 Barrett, J. and T. Pitman. *Pregnancy and Birth: The best evidence.* Toronto: Key Porter Books, 1999.

15 Wiley Lorente, Carole. "Mother of midwifery." *Vegetarian Times*, July 1995.

16 Harper, B. *Gentle Birth Choices.* Rochester: Healing Arts Press, 1994.

BIRTHING NATURALLY WITH A DOULA

1 Sheila Kitzinger, 2001, "Awake, aware—and action" *Birth-Issues in Perinatal Care*, (September) 28.3, <http://www.sheilakitzinger.com/BIRTH-Awake.htm>.

BIRTHING NATURALLY UNASSISTED

1 Michel Odent and Christine Hauch, 1989, *Entering the World: The De-Medicalization of Childbirth.* London: Marion Boyars Publishers.

2 Frederick Leboyer, 1995, *Birth Without Violence.* (Dorset, UK: Element Books Ltd).

BIRTHING NATURALLY THE FIRST OR THE NEXT TIME

1 R. J. Jarret, J. Castro-Soares, A. Dornhorst, and R. Beard, 1997, "Should we screen for gestational diabetes?" *British Medical Journal (BMJ)* 315; 736–9.

2 S. Kilpatrick, 1995, "Unlike pre-eclampsia, gestational hypertension is not associated with increased neonatal and maternal morbidity except abruptions," *SPO abstracts, Am. J. Obstet. Gynecol*, 419; 376.

3 O. Koller, R. Sandvei, and N. Sagen, 1980, "High hemoglobin levels during pregnancy and fetal risk," *Int. J. Gynaecol. Obstet,* 18:53–6.

4 See P. Steer, M.A. Alam, J. Wadsworth, and A. Welch, 1995, "Relation between maternal haemoglobin concentration and birth weight in different ethnic groups," *BMJ,* 310; 489–91.

5 Michel Odent, 2002, *The farmer and the obstetrician.* London: Free Association Books), p. 130.

6 See <www.birthpsychology.com/primalhealth> for a series of useful articles.

7 Pitocin is the synthetic hormone used to induce labor. The natural hormone involved in labor progression is called oxytocin.

8 For more on this birth story, see Claudia Villeneuve's birth story, p. 115.

9 VBAC stands for vaginal birth after caesarean.

10 Dr. Odent shared some telling anecdotes about successful midwives, notably one from Italy who had a very labor-intensive enema-making task for the father. Cutting thin strips of soap off a block, boiling them to a smooth melt, and then letting the mixture cool down was a process that usually took longer than the baby's birth and served as a good distraction for the father. Dr. Odent calls such an activity a "couvade," which means "hatching" or a task such as boiling water, that helps a man to feel useful during the birthing process and keeps him out of the way, to put it bluntly.

11 Reinekke Lengelle worked as a clinical chemist for twenty-five years in a large urban hospital in The Netherlands.

12 With a nod to doula Annemarie van Oploo.

13 See Pam England's book with the same title.

14 See Pam England.

15 Laborland as described by Pam England is the place a woman goes to during labor to cope with pain. It is an endorphin-induced "trance" in which a laboring woman may look distant or respond out of character.

16 When someone close to the laboring woman becomes alarmed (and releases adrenaline) this can affect the laboring woman by triggering her own flight/fight response. As adrenaline works directly opposed to hormones like oxytocin that promote labor, it is important that the woman and those present at birth stay calm.

17 See books by the American author Debbie Ford and work by the renowned Italian psychiatrist Robert Assagioli, founder of psychosynthesis, who did groundbreaking work in this area.

18 See Reinekke Lengelle, 2001, "An early miscarriage," *Birth Issues,* Fall 20 issue.

19 See Byron Katie and Stephen Mitchell, 2003, *Loving what is: Four questions that can change your life,* (New York: Three Rivers Press). For more information also see her Web site at <www.thework.org>.

References

Birthing Naturally with a Midwife

Alberta Health Disciplines Board. Investigation of Midwifery Final Report and Recommendations. Edmonton: Alberta Health, Feb. 1991.

Association for Safe Alternatives in Childbirth (ASAC). *Midwives: What Canadian women deserve*, 1998. [media package]

Arms, A. *Immaculate Deception II: Myth, Magic & Birth*, Berkeley, CA: Celestial Arts, 1994.

Banks, A. C. *Birth Chairs, Midwives, and Medicine.* Jackson: University Press of Mississippi, 1999.

Botting, S. "Safety and midwifery care in Alberta." *Birthing*, Summer 1998.

Buhler, L. et al. "Prenatal care: a comparative evaluation of nurse-midwives and family physicians." *Canadian Medical Association Journal.* 139 (1998): 397–403.

Douglas, Ann. *The mother of all pregnancy books: An all-canadian guide to conception, birth and everything in between.* Toronto: CDG Books Canada Inc., 2000.

Durand, M. A. "The safety of home birth: The farm study." *American Journal of Public Health.* 82 (1992): 450–52.

England, P. *The truth about childbirth.* Nov. 21, 2004, Edmonton, Alberta. [lecture]

England, P. and Horowitz, R. *Birthing from Within*. Albuquerque, NM: Partera Press, 1998.

Goer, H. *Obstetrical Myths versus Research Realities*. Westport, CT: Bergin & Garvey, 1995.

Greenhalgh, J. Personal communication. 30 March 2004.

Hawkings, M and Knox, S. *The Midwifery Option*. Toronto: HarperCollins, 2003.

Janssen, P. A. et al. "Outcomes of planned home births after regulation of midwifery in British Columbia." *Canadian Medical Association Journal*. 166 (Feb. 2002): 3. <http://www.cmaj.ca/cgi/content/full/166/3/315>.

Marck, P. "For home birth moms, there's no other way." *The Edmonton Journal*, 13 May 1995.

National Association of Childbearing Centers (NACC) <http://www2.birthcenters.org/faqbirthcenters>.

Obstetrical Working Group of the National Health Insurance Board of the Netherlands. *Obstetric Manual* (English translation, abridged version), 2000. <http://europe.obgyn.net/nederland/default.asp?page=/nederland/richtlijnen/vademecum_eng>.

Odent, M. "Can humanity survive the industrialization of childbirth?" Edmonton: ASAC, 2003. [CD set]

Odent, M. *Primal Health*. East Sussex ,UK: Clareview Books, 2002.

Tyson, H. "Outcomes of 1001 midwife-attended home births in Toronto, 1983–1988." Birth 18 (March 1991): 1.

van Olphen-Fehr, J. *Diary of a Midwife*. Westport, CT: Bergin & Garvey, 1998.

Walker, N. *A guide to pregnancy, birth and postpartum*. Edmonton: Passages Midwifery, 2000.

Birthing Naturally with a Physician

Barrett, Joyce and Pitman, Teresa. 1999. *Pregnancy and birth: The best evidence*. Toronto, Ont: Key Porter Books.

Diamond, Susan L. 1998. *Hard labor*. New York: Forge.

Gaskin, Ina May. 2003. *Ina May's guide to childbirth*. New York: Bantam.

Goer, Henci and Wheeler, Rhonda. 1999. *The thinking woman's guide to a better birth*. New York: Perigee Books.

Korte, Diana and Scaer, Roberta. 1992. *A good birth, a safe birth.* Boston: Harvard Common Press.

Leboyer, Frederick. 1995. *Birth without Violence.* Dorset, UK: Element Books Ltd.

Odent, Michel. 1994. *Birth reborn.* Medford, NJ: Birth Works, Inc.

Sears, William and Martha. 1994. *The birth book.* New York: Little, Brown.

Simkin, Penny, Whalley, Janet, and Keppler, Ann. 2003. *Pregnancy, childbirth and the newborn: The complete guide.* New York: Simon & Schuster.

Wolf, Naomi. 2003. *Misconceptions: truth, lies, and the unexpected on the journey to motherhood.* New York: Anchor Books/Doubleday.

BIRTHING NATURALLY THE FIRST OR NEXT TIME

England, Pam and Horowitz, Rob. 1998. *Birthing from within.* Albuquerque, NM: Partera Press.

Gottman, John and Silver, Nan. 2000. *The seven principles for making marriage work.* New York: Three Rivers Press.

Katie, Byron and Mitchell, Stephen. 2003. *Loving what is: Four questions that can change your life.* New York: Three Rivers Press.

Lengelle, Reinekke. 2001. "An early miscarriage." *Birth Issues,* Fall.

Northrup, Christiane. 2002. *Women's bodies, women's wisdom.* Revised edition. New York: Bantam Books.

Odent, Michel. 1999. *The scientification of love.* London, UK: Free Association Books.

Odent, Michel. 2002. *The farmer and the obstetrician.* London, UK: Free Association Books.

Pennebaker, James. 1997. *Opening up: The healing power of expressing emotions.* Reprint edition. New York: The Guilford Press.

Additional Resources

⁓

PUBLICATIONS

Arms, Suzanne. 1975. *Immaculate deception*. Boston: Houghton Mifflin.

Buhler, L. et al. 1998. "Prenatal care: a comparative evaluation of nurse-midwives and family physicians." *Canadian Medical Association Journal*. 139: 397–403.

Carson Banks, Amanda. 1999. *Birth chairs, midwives and medicine*. Jackson: University Press of Mississippi.

Davis, Elizabeth, Arms, Suzanne, and Harrison, Linda. 1997. *Heart & hands: a midwife's guide to pregnancy & birth*. Berkeley, CA: Celestial Arts.

Davis-Floyd, Robbie E. 2004. *Birth as an American rite of passage*. Berkeley, CA: University of California.

Douglas, Ann. 2000. *The mother of all pregnancy books: An all-Canadian guide to conception, birth and everything in between*. Toronto: CDG Books Inc.

Gaskin, Ina May. 2002. *Spiritual midwifery*. Summertown, TN: Book Publishing Company.

Goer, Henci. 1995. *Obstetrical myths versus research realities*. Westport, CT: Bergin & Garvey.

Harper, Barbara and Arms, Suzanne (photographer). 1994. *Gentle birth choices: A guide to making informed decisions about birthing centers, birth attendants, water birth, home birth, hospital birth*. Rochester, VT: Healing Art Press.

Kennell, John, and Klaus, Marshall and Phyllis. 1993. *Mothering the mother: How a doula can help you have a shorter, easier and healthier birth.* Boston: Addison-Wesley.

Kitzinger, Sheila. 1991. *Homebirth.* London: Dk Publishers.

Kitzinger, Sheila. 2000. *Rediscovering birth.* London: Little, Brown.

Kitzinger, Sheila. 2003. *The complete book of pregnancy and childbirth.* New York: Knopf.

Klaus, Marshall, Kennell, John and Klaus, Phyllis. 2002. *The doula book: How a trained labor companion can help you have a shorter, easier, and healthier birth.* Cambridge, MA: Perseus Books.

La Leche League. 2003. *The breastfeeding answer book.* La Leche League International.

Liedloff, Jean. 1986. *The continuum concept: In search of happiness lost.* Boston: Addison-Wesley.

Newman, Jack and Pitman, Theresa. 2000. *The ultimate breastfeeding book of answers.* Roseville, CA: Prima Lifestyles.

Noble, Elizabeth, with Sorger, Leo. 2003. *Having twins—and more: A parent's guide to multiple pregnancy, birth, and early childhood.* Boston: Mariner Books.

Odent, Michel. 1989. *Entering the world: The de-medicalization of childbirth.* London, UK: Marion Boyars Publishers.

Odent, Michel. 2002. *Primal Health.* East Sussex, UK: Clareview Books.

Odent, Michel. Primal Health newsletter <www.birthpsychology.com/primalhealth/>.

Perez, Paulina, and Snedeker, Cheryl. 1994. *Special women: The role of the professional labor assistant.* International Childbirth Education Association.

Shanley, Laura Kaplan. 1993. *Unassisted childbirth.* Westport, CT: Bergin & Garvey.

Simkin, Penny. 1989. *The birth partner: Everything you need to know to help a woman through childbirth.* National Book Network.

Sinclair, Patti. 2002. *Motherhood as a spiritual practice.* Edmondton, AB: Motherspace Unlimited Publishing.

Storch, J. 1982. *Patient rights: Ethical and legal issues in health care and nursing.* Toronto: McGraw Hill Ryerson.

Tonder Hansen, Maren. 1997. *Mother mysteries.* Boston: Shambhala.

van Olphen-Fehr, J. 1998. *Diary of a midwife.* Westport, CT: Bergin & Garvey.

Verny, Thomas and Kelly, John. 1988. *The secret life of the unborn child.* New York: Dell.

Wainer Cohen, Nancy, and Estner, Lois. 1983. *Silent knife: Cesarean prevention and vaginal birth after cesarean (VBAC).* Westport, CT: Bergin & Garvey.

Wirth, Frederick. 2001. *Prenatal Parenting.* New York: ReganBooks.

ORGANIZATIONS

Association for Safe Alternatives in Childbirth (ASAC)
Main Post Office Box 1197
Edmonton, AB
Canada, T5J 2M4
Phone: (780) 425-7993
Web site: <www.asac.ab.ca>

Association of Labor Assistants and Childbirth Educators (ALACE)
PO Box 390436
Cambridge, MA 02139
Phone: (888) 222-5223
Web site: <www.alace.org>

Canadian Association of Midwives (CAM)
#207-2051 McCallum Rd.
Abbotsford, BC
Canada, V2S 3N5
Web site: <http://members.rogers.com/canadianmidwives/>

Childbirth and Postpartum Professional Association (CAPPA)
PO Box 491448
Lawrenceville, GA 30049
Phone: (888) MY-CAPPA
Web site: <www.cappa.net/labordo.asp>

Doulas of North America (DONA)
PO Box 626
Jasper, IN 47547
Phone: (206) 324-5440
Web site: <www.DONA.com>

The Farm Midwives
Phone: (931) 964-2472
Web site: <www.thefarm.org>

International Childbirth Education Association (ICEA)
PO Box 20048
Minneapolis, MN 55420
Phone: (612) 854-8660
Web site: <www.icea.org.>

Lamaze International
2025 M Street, Suite 800
Washington, DC 20036-3309
Phone: (800) 368-4404
Web site: <www.lamaze-childbirth.com>

Maternity Wise
Maternity Center Association
281 Park Avenue South, 5th Floor
New York, NY 10010
Phone: (212) 777-5000
Web site: <www.maternitywise.org>

Midwifery Alliance of North America (MANA)
375 Rockbridge Road, Suite 172-313
Lilburn, Georgia 30047
Phone: (888) 923-6262
Web site: <www.mana.org>

Acknowledgments

⌒

T<small>HE</small> A<small>SSOCIATION FOR</small> Safe Alternatives in Childbirth (ASAC) is a
nonprofit organization in Canada that has been sharing information
about natural childbirth for twenty-five years. You can read more about ASAC
at <www.asac.ab.ca>. Besides offering information nights, play groups, and a
library specializing in pregnancy, birth, and parenting, ASAC publishes *Birth
Issues* magazine. Each issue of *Birth Issues* contains a few birth stories. There are
about a hundred birth stories on the Web site and more are posted every few
months.

To share birth stories and motivations for natural childbirth, ASAC members decided to put together *Adventures in Natural Childbirth.* A team solicited
birth stories from across North America; collected 130 stories; read them,
reread them, and read them again; selected thirty-nine for inclusion in the book
and posted most of the rest on the ASAC Web site; and wrote introductory
chapters for each section. We also created some original illustrations that do
more than decorate the book; they demonstrate methods of coping and optimal
positions during pregnancy and labor.

I could not and did not create *Adventures in Natural Childbirth* without the
work of many others. Members of the *Adventures in Natural Childbirth* team are

Dawn Freeman, Deanne Frere, Sally Kucher, Reinekke Lengelle, Cathy McMillan, Christina Otterstrom-Cedar, Dana Ovcharenko, Sue Robins, Connie Schneider, Patti Sinclair, Annemarie van Oploo, Claudia Villeneuve, Elizabeth Wall, and Deborah Webb. Liz, Deanne, Sue, Claudia, Dawn, Reinekke, Cathy, and I chose the stories to be included in the book. Reinekke, Christina, Claudia, Dawn, and Annemarie researched and wrote the introductory essays for each section. Cathy, a professional illustrator, created the illustrations for the inside pages. Claudia, a professional doula, provided the captions. Dawn, Patti, Dana, and Deborah performed the first round of editing. Deb also provided design concepts for the cover and suggestions for the layout of the inside pages. Reinekke and Annemarie prepared the comprehensive glossary of terms related to pregnancy and birth. Dawn played a big role, and I want to give her a special thank-you; I felt her presence with me as I worked on the book. I did the final editing and take responsibility for any errors or omissions in the book (except, of course, if you take the book's statements or stories as advice without consulting with your care provider).

A few more thank-yous are in order. I want to thank my husband, Bryan, and daughter, Allison, for their patience and support, especially when I brought work with me on vacation, more than once. No doubt other members of the team also owe debts of gratitude to their family members, so here is an official "thank-you" for accommodating this project into your lives.

Index